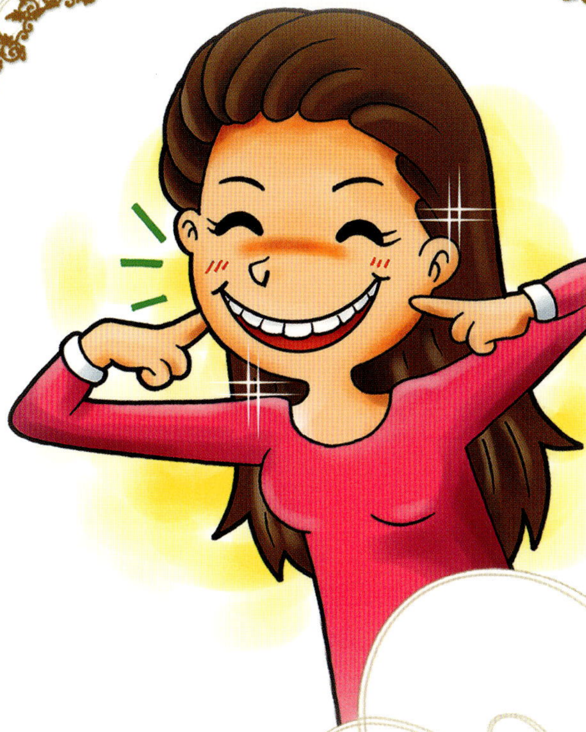

A Dentist Can Make You More Beautiful!

By Dr. Ho-Sung, Lew, D.D.S., PH.D.
Orthodontic Specialist

MYUNG MUN PUBLISHING

Author's Comments

Profile of the Author

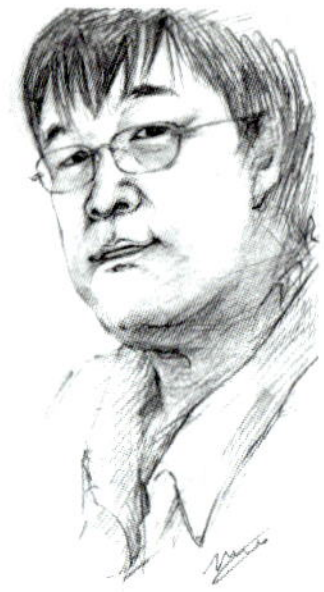

Ho-Sung, Lew D.D.S., Ph.D.
Orthodontic Specialist
Woong Dental Clinic, Suwon, Korea
Telephone: 82-31-243-2828
Fax: 82-31-255-2875
E-mail: orthopia@hanmail.net

1996~Present:

Private Practice as an Orthodontist, Korea
Member of Korean Orthodontist Society
Head of Millennium Flute Choir, Korea
The Author of 11 Books Including Several Essays

1995~96:

Assistant Professor,
Department of Orthodontics, School of Dentistry,
Tokushima University, Japan

1991~95:

Received Ph. D. from
Graduate School of Dentistry, Tokushima University, Japan

1987~91:

Private General Practice
Mugug-ri Kumwang-up, Choongbuk Province, Korea

1981~87:

Received D.D.S. from
College of Dentistry, Dankook University, Chonan, Korea

1977~79:

Served in the Korean Army as a Medic

1976:

Entered Korea University, Seoul, Korea

Profiles of the Translators

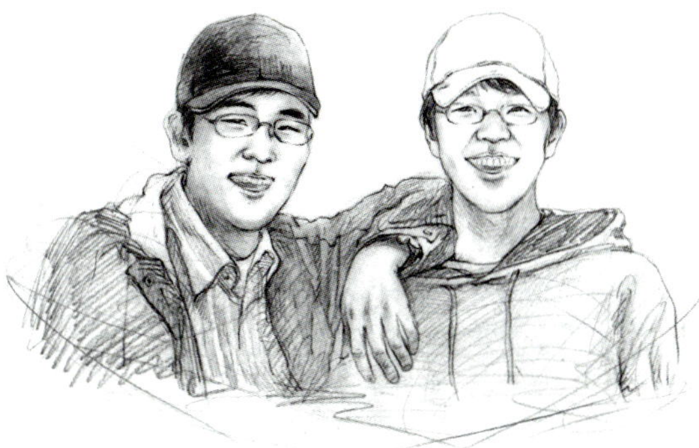

Jung-Hwan, Lew

Born in Seoul, Korea, 1986.
Entered Simon Fraser University, Vancouver, Canada.
Transferred to the Matsumoto Dental University, Japan.
Currently in the 5th Grade.

Gil-Hwan, Lew

Born in Seoul, Korea, 1989.
3rd Grade, Department of Chemistry,
University of British Columbia, Vancouver, Canada

To the Readers

Thirty years have passed since I entered the School of Dentistry and started learning dentistry. During those years, I made copious notes of information that I felt would be helpful to my future patients who would receive orthodontic treatments. I also took many photographs of treatment procedures and prepared drawings which I put into this book to help readers gain a better understanding of what orthodontics mean. Although this book may lack in certain aspects, it is the crystallization of my prolonged efforts.

These days people gain information about orthodontics through newspapers, radios, magazines, television and other forms of mass media including internet. Unfortunately, however, because of the limited knowledge they obtain in the field of orthodontic treatment, many people make the mistake of jumping to their own conclusions.

As a result, many people miss the proper treatment period or do not visit an orthodontist for a simple treatment due to neglection. Also, many people believe that orthodontic treatments is very expensive and consequently defer necessary treatment after adolescence. Some people think that teeth must be extracted to treat badly aligned teeth. But, in fact, all of these are not true.

I will be highly gratified if there is at least one person who receives treatment at a proper time because of this book and if this book helps clear up any misunderstandings between the patient and the orthodontist regarding treatment procedures.

I would like to thank my parents and an elder brother for the support and encouragement they have given me so far. I would also like to mention that the loving support of my two sons, Jung-Hwan and Gil-Hwan, plus my wife always has remained the major source of inspiration and stamina to me.

June 10, 2012
Ho-Sung Lew

Acknowledgements

I would like to express my deepest gratitude
to Professor Terushige Kawata,
in addition to my parents, wife and two sons,
whose untold sacrifices
made my successful career as an orthodontist possible.

Main Points of This Book

From the beginning of civilizations, clear bright eyes and good alignment of teeth were considered as conditions for being beautiful. Our ancestors have considered good teeth alignment as an important factor in determining facial beauty.

Badly aligned teeth also lead to various forms of dental diseases such as dental caries, gum diseases, and malocclusions. It is a well-known fact that if the teeth of both upper and lower jaws have no crowdings and function in good harmony, incidence of dental diseases such as decayed teeth(dental caries), and gum diseases(periodontitis) are greatly decreased.

Receiving orthodontic treatments will not only straighten the teeth alignment, but also will normalize the functions in the oral cavity by changing the way you talk, chew, and swallow. In addition, it will also improve your self-esteem.

Table of Contents

Author's Comments

Table of Contents

III. Breast Feeding and Nursing Bottle

IV. Occlusions

V. Various Kinds of Malocclusions

I. A History of Orthodontics

1. Neatly Aligned Teeth Determine One's Beauty

A. Plastic Surgery

B. Orthodontic Treatment

C. Formation of Human Teeth

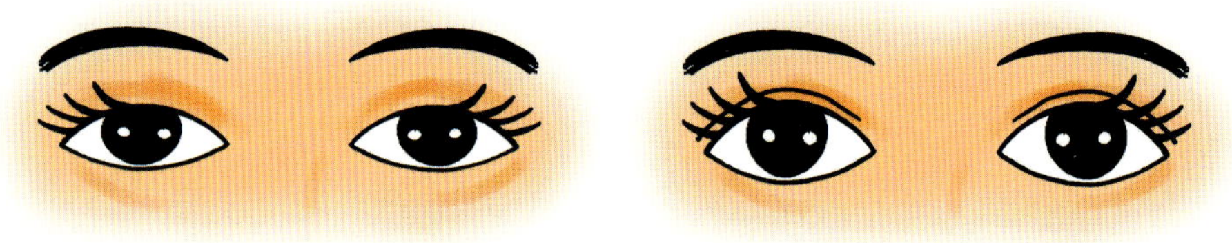

A. Plastic Surgery

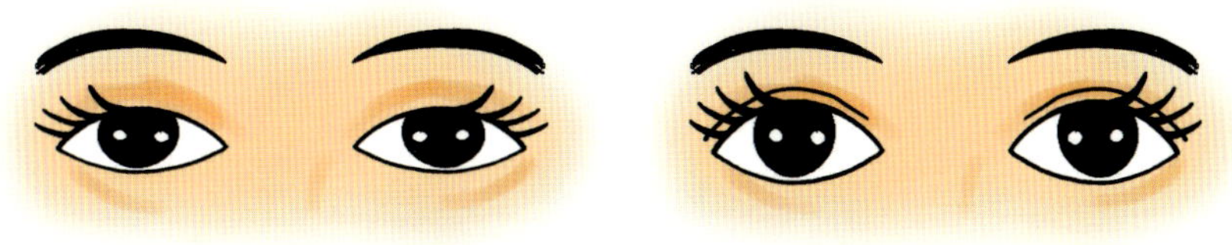

double eye lid surgery(Asian blepharoplasty)

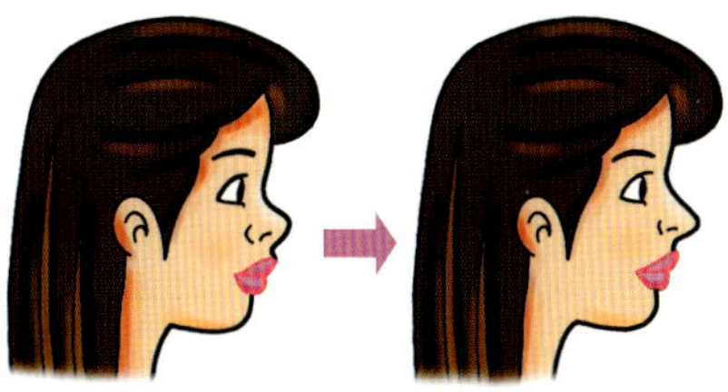

nose surgery for esthetics(rhinoplasty)

From the ancient times, our ancestors believed that beauty stems from clear and pretty eyes, lovely facial expressions, and a neatly aligned set of teeth.

Plastic surgeries for eyes and nose are similar to orthodontic treatments in the sense that they are performed to make the face more attractive. Even though one receives a plastic surgery for eyes, this person will not necessarily have better eye sight. Furthermore, one who receives a nose surgery for improving the nasal appearance will not be able to breathe better nor have a keener sense of smell.

B. Orthodontic Treatment

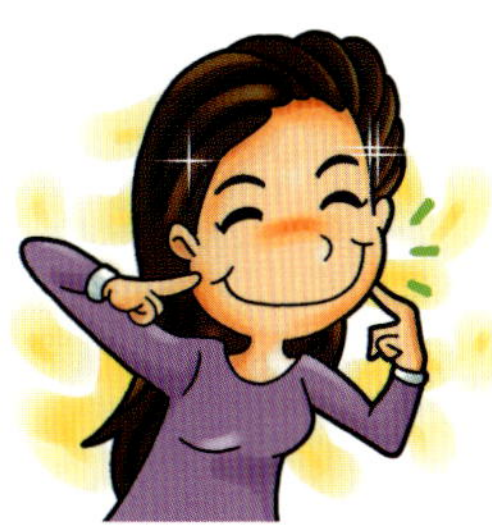

A person receiving orthodontic treatment will not only have a good alignment of teeth, but will also be able to speak, chew, and swallow more efficiently. In addition, the patient will have a better appearance afterwards.

Therefore, receiving orthodontic treatment will enable one to look more attractive and normalize the oral functions. For these reasons, orthodontic treatments differ from plastic surgeries.

C. Formation of Human Teeth

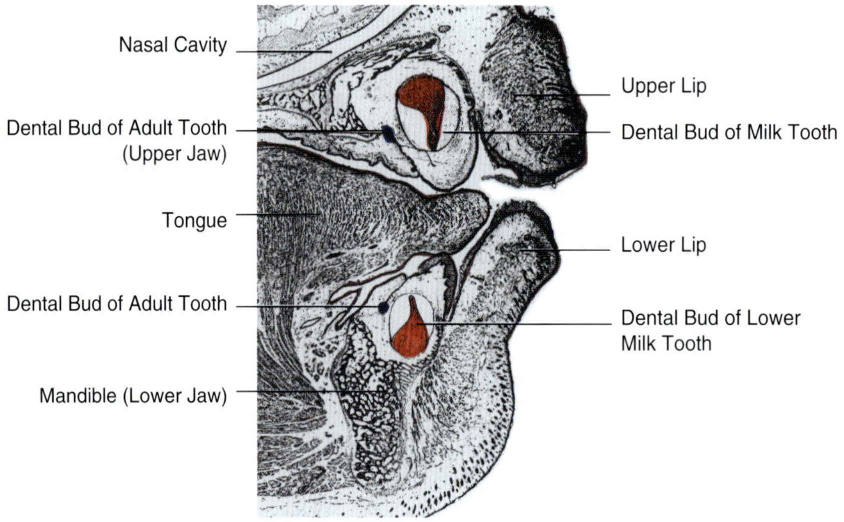

Human fetus 200mm, about 18 weeks (modified photo from S. N. Bhaskar Orban's Oral histology and embryology, The C.V. Mosby, 1980)

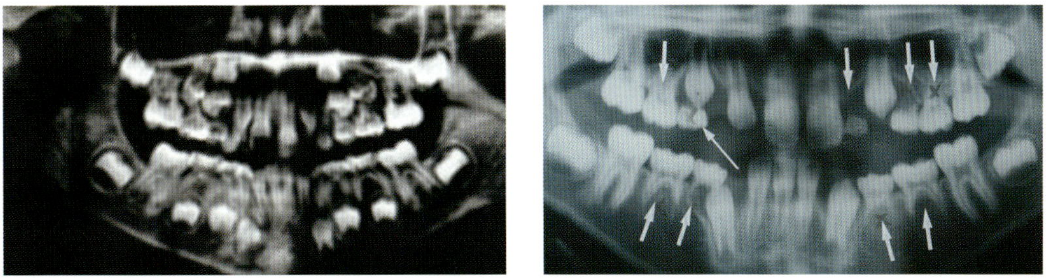

Permanent teeth are growing underneath the milk teeth(left). The person in the right photo is almost the same age as the one in the left photo. Arrows show congenital missing of adult teeth. There are no dental buds corresponding to the adult teeth.

We are apt to think that the teeth are made after birth. Dental buds which will become teeth in the future are already formed during the period of 4~6 weeks of pregnancy. So number, shape, size of the teeth irrespective of permanent and deciduous(milk) are already decided during the early period of pregnancy, and can not be changed afterwards.

After birth, human body continues to grow as time goes by, but the size and the numbers of teeth themselves do not change at all. Only the shape of the root of individual tooth changes until it reaches its mature stage.

2. Orthodontic Appliances of Prehistoric Ages

A. Etruscan and Phoenician Remains

B. Fixing the Teeth by Wire

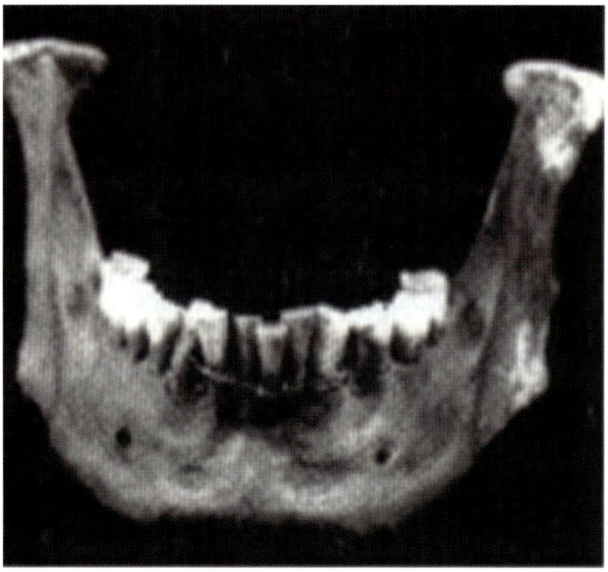

A. Etruscan and Phoenician Remains

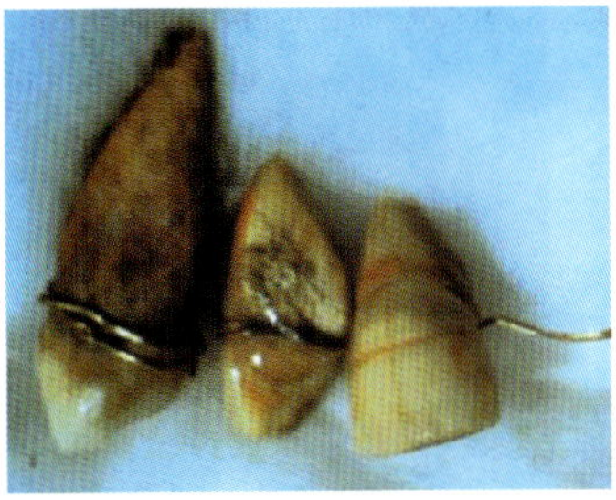

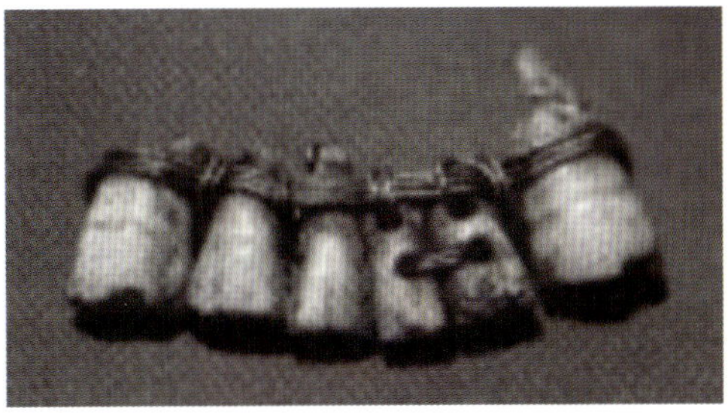

Remains of the prehistoric ages such as Maya and Phoenicia

Although in primitive times, well-designed devices that seemingly designed to align the teeth are being found in anciently civilized areas such as Etruria, Phoenicia, Greece, and the Mayans of Mexico.

Poorly aligned teeth have always been considered a problem for ages, and the effort to treat a badly aligned teeth has been attempted since at least 1,000 B.C.

B. Fixing the Teeth by Wire

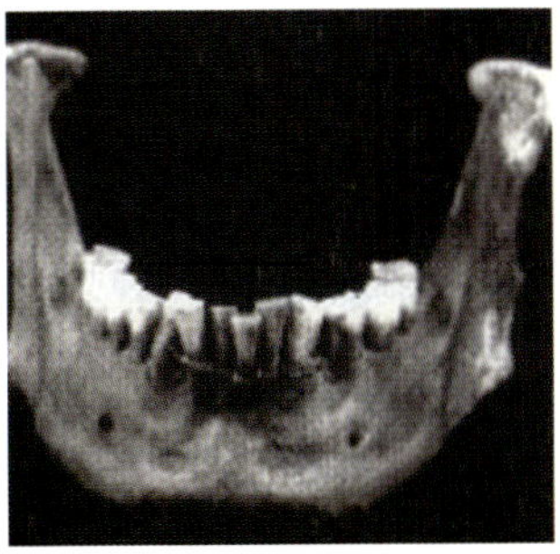

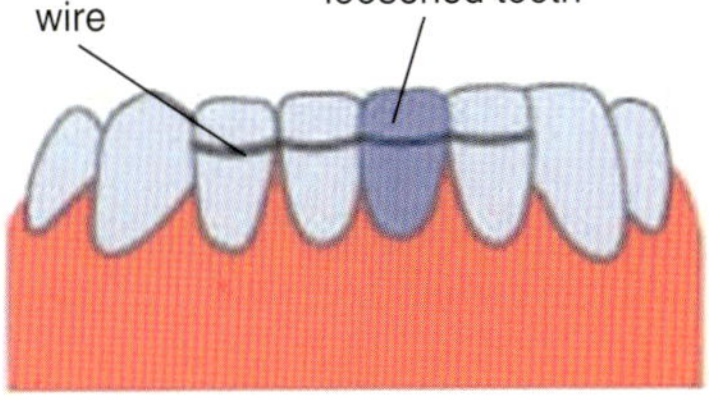

wire fixation

The left illustration is supposed to be remains from ancient Greece, 300 B.C.. Because of poorly aligned teeth, a gum disease might have been resulted and caused the teeth to be loosened. Therefore, a gold wire was ligated for fixing the loosened teeth. The technique used in this illustration was very precise. Presently loosened teeth are fixed by wire just the same manner as shown in the right illustration.

3. Life Conditions of Prehistoric Man

A. Hard and Coarse Food Stuffs

B. Changes in Dietary Habit

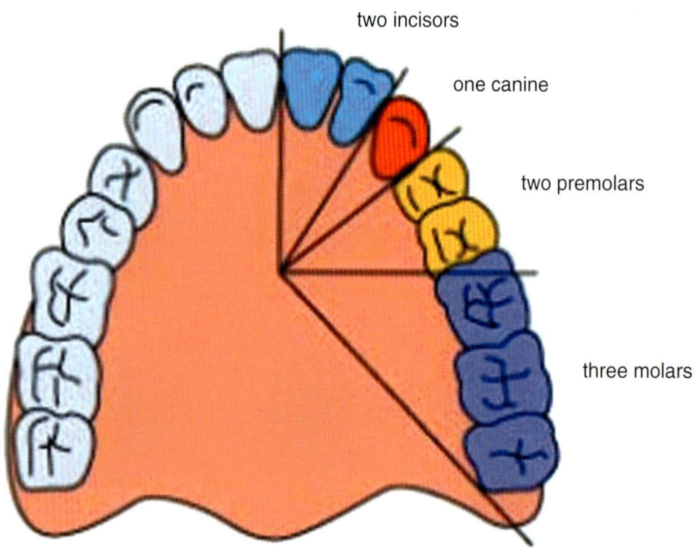

A. Hard and Coarse Food Materials

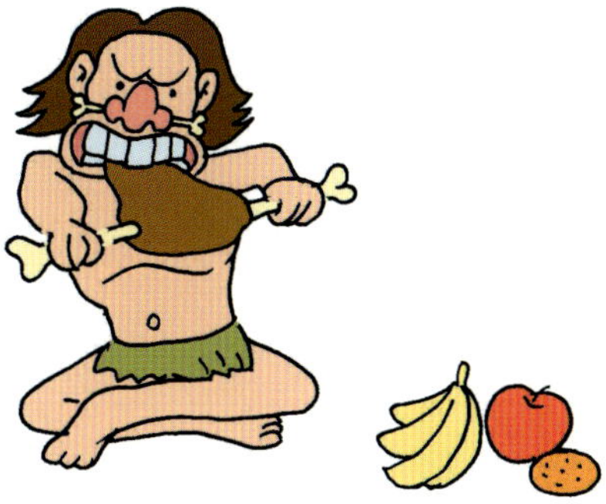

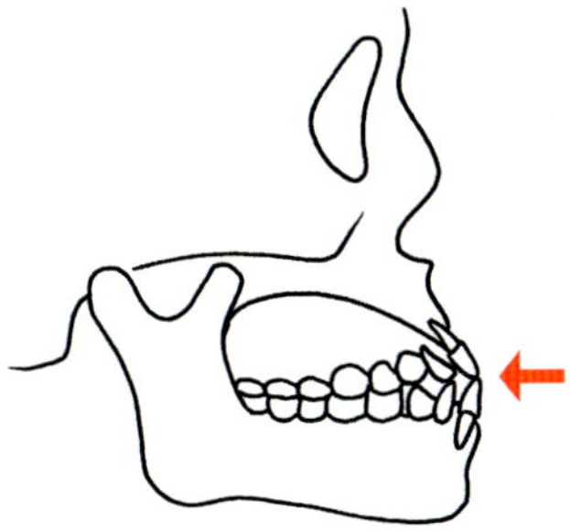

Upper and lower front teeth contact edge-to-edge like tweezers.

Compared to human beings living 10,000 years ago, people today generally have worse alignments of teeth. As humans began to use fire, food was roasted or boiled and became softer. As a result, a need for large-sized teeth and strong jaws was decreased.

Cavemen had to eat raw meat, hard fruits, and nuts in order to survive in their harsh environments. In order to do so, they had to have strong jaw bones and large-sized teeth to eat the hard and tough food materials. Cavemen's front teeth were contacted edge-to-edge like tweezers and they had very large and strong jaws. These shapes of the jaws and teeth were ideal in chewing hard and tough food materials.

B. Changes in Dietary Habit

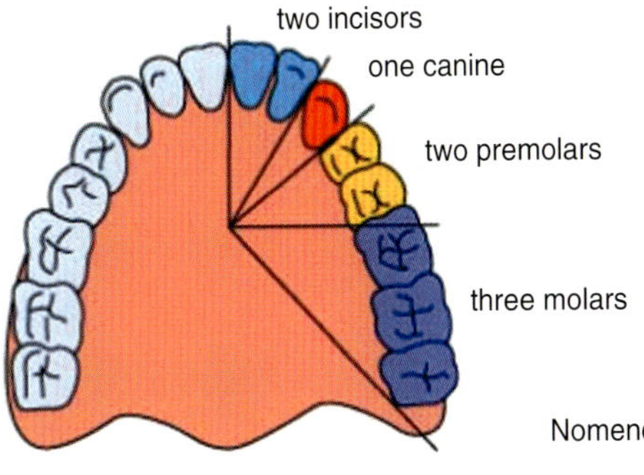

Nomenclature of Adult Teeth

As civilizations progressed, people began to eat refined and cooked foods. As a matter of course, the need to chew or bite down hard food materials became unnecessary. This led them to have smaller and weaker jaws.

In addition, due to evolution, people today have a smaller number of teeth compared to humans of the far past. The fact that some modern peoples do not have wisdom teeth, premolars, or lateral incisors in their mouths, proves that this evolutionary process is still taking place.

4. Evolutionary Changes in the Shape of Head and Neck

A. Head and Jaw Bones

B. Alveolar and Basal Bone of Jaw

C. Modern People's Front Teeth

D. Mandibular Body

E. Profile Changes

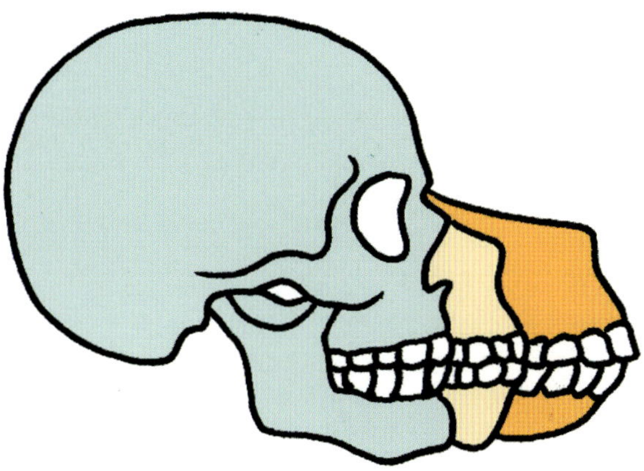

A. Head and Jaw Bones

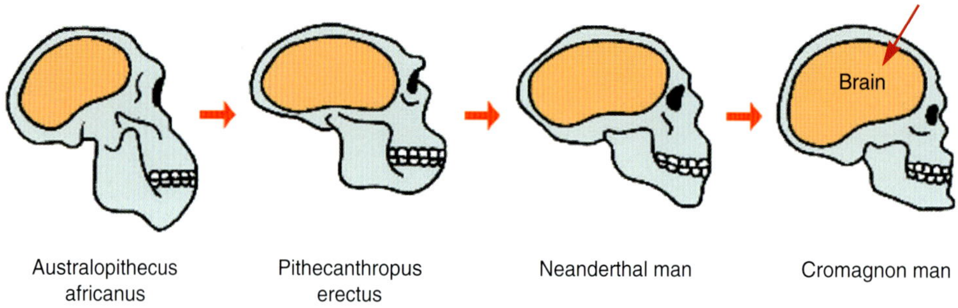

Through analyzing the skulls of people lived in the past, it is evident that evolution had a great effect on the shape of human head and face. To fight against wild beasts or eat tough food materials, people living thousands of years ago had developed strong jaws and cheek bones.

Ancient human skulls used to resemble those of monkeys, but as time progressed, the shape of head and face slowly changed. The size of jaws and cheek bones decreased, whereas brains of human beings became larger.

B. Alveolar and Basal Bone of Jaw

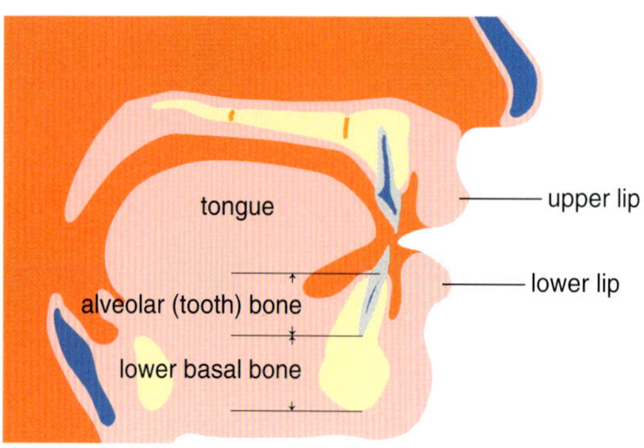

A jaw bone consists of two parts, that is called alveolar bone, and the bone beneath is called basal bone.

An alveolar bone is the thickened ridge of bone that contains the tooth sockets on the basal bone. That is, alveolar bone encases the root of individual tooth on the basal bones. In humans, the tooth-bearing bones are the maxilla(upper jaw) and the mandible(lower jaw). The anatomical texture of alveolar bone and basal bone is very different from each other.

Primitive cavemen had a bony thickening on the front of the lower jaw called simian shelf. Its function is to reinforce the jaw. It also has the effect of considerable reduced movement of the tongue by restricting the area available for muscles.

As the biting frequencies diminished, the alveolar bone began to shift backwards. However, the location of the basal bone remains unchanged.

Thus, the dividing line between the alveolar and the basal bone began to appear. So, when you push the part beneath the lower lip, you will feel a section that has sunk in. This is a proof that an evolution has taken place to change the lower part of human face.

C. Modern People's Front Teeth

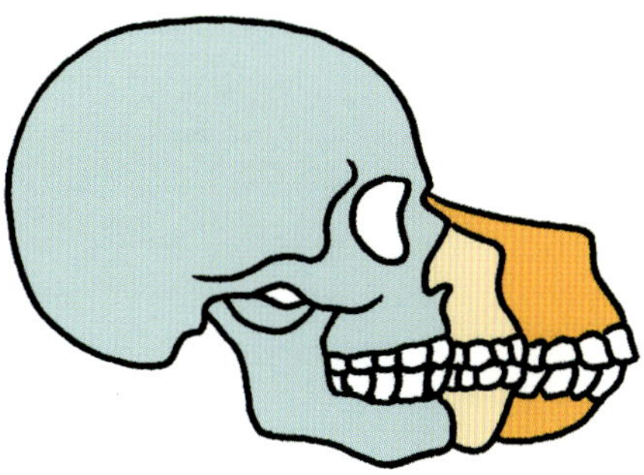

Evolutionary Change of Human Face

Most modern people's front teeth of upper jaw cover the front teeth of lower jaw. This is because the entire set of teeth, so called dentition, of the lower jaw have regressed back.

D. Mandibular Body

The horizontal, horseshoe-shaped portion of the lower jaw which continues on either side backward and upward into the ramus is known as a mandibular body. As civilization progressed, the entire length of lower jaw, called mandibular body, became shorter, resulted in insufficient space for wisdom tooth. Thus, modern people suffer from complications caused by frequent impaction of wisdom teeth.

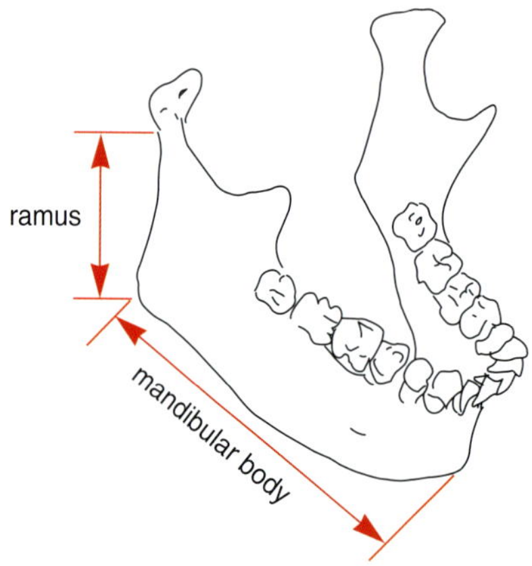

horseshoe-shaped mandible

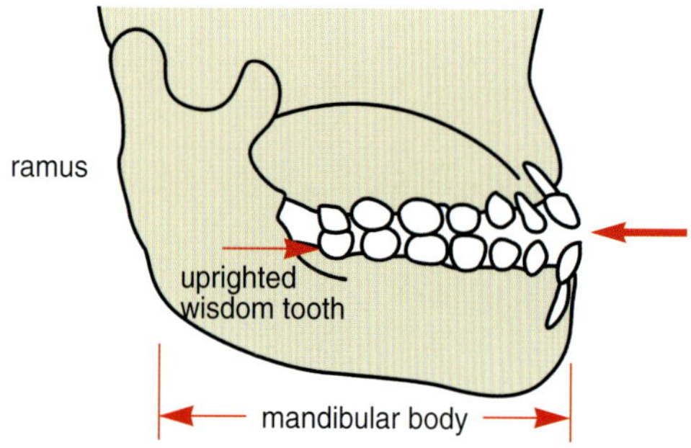

primitive man

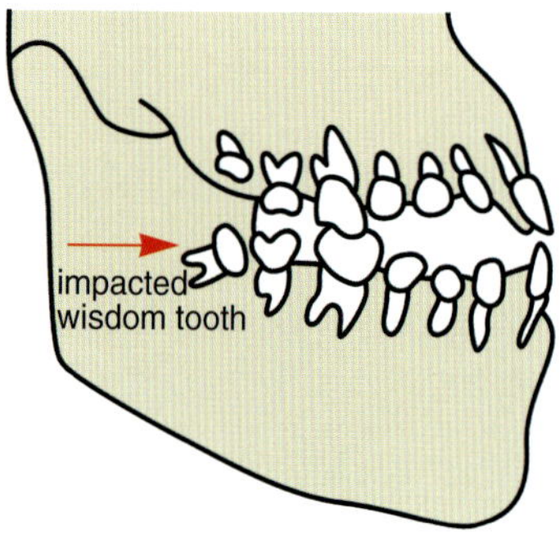

modern people

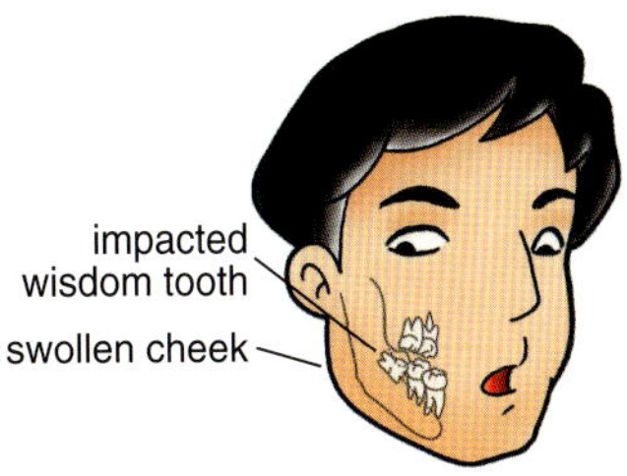

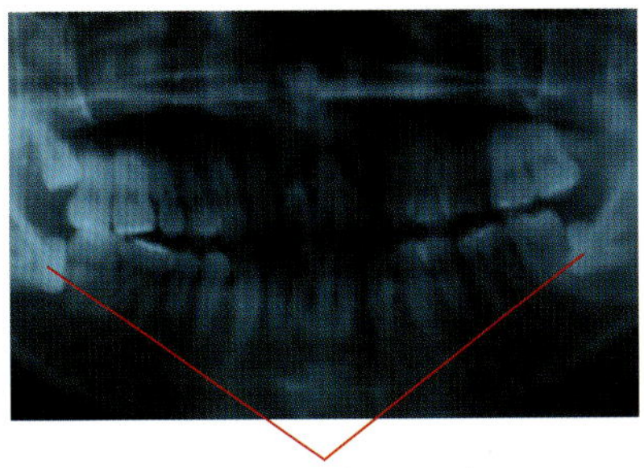

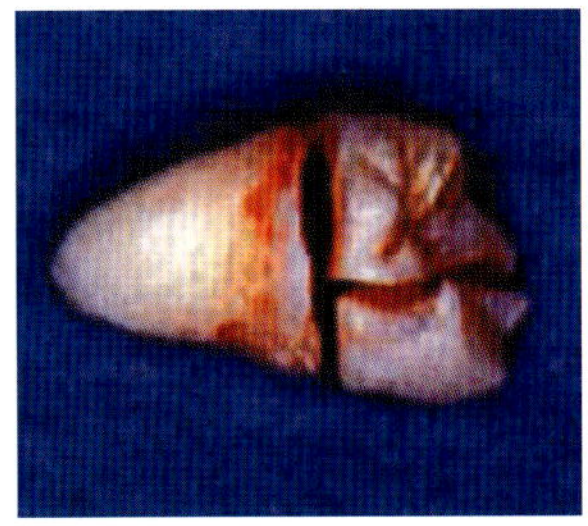

Swollen cheek caused by impacted wisdom tooth. It is recognized by x-ray, and removed by surgery

E. Profile Changes

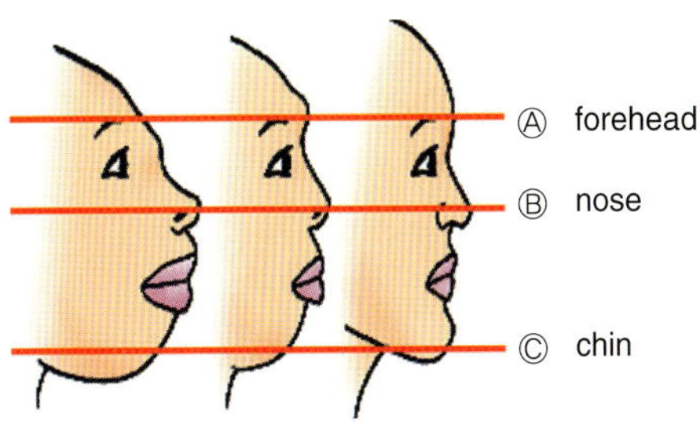

Even though the shape of the head and neck region has changed as the time elapsed, the points of the forehead (A), nose (B), and chin (C) do not differ in locations. In other words, the points where the eyes, nose, and lips are located remains the same.

Because the alveolar bones of upper and lower jaws have sunk in, this leads to a relatively higher nose and the chin pointing outwards.

II. Alignment of the Upper and Lower Teeth

5. The Western Perceptions of the Alignment of Teeth

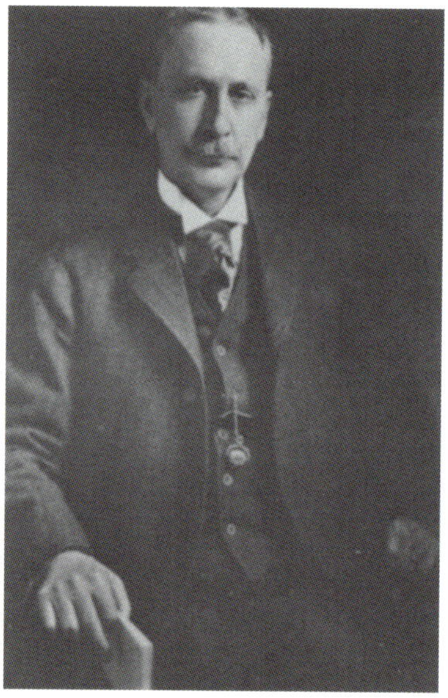

Edward H. Angle, the father of modern Orthodontics
(Proffit WR. Contemporary Orthodontics, 3rd. ed. St. Louis, 2000, Mosby-Yearbook)

When judging the attractiveness of a person, we tend to look at the eyes, nose, and lips, along with the alignment of their teeth. If one has a bad alignment of teeth, this could have a negative effect on the facial appearance and the harmony of the human body.

The study of "ORTHODONTICS" was originated in Europe, and entering this century, its rapid progress has taken place in the United States. Westerners consider neatly aligned teeth as a sign of good health.

Therefore, parents of Western countries pay a deep attention to their children's teeth alignment from an early age. Before puberty, most of the children receive orthodontic treatments. Almost the whole adults living in Western countries have good alignment of teeth not because they were born with them, but because they have received orthodontic treatments in earlier stages of their lives.

6. Practicing the Orthodontic Treatment

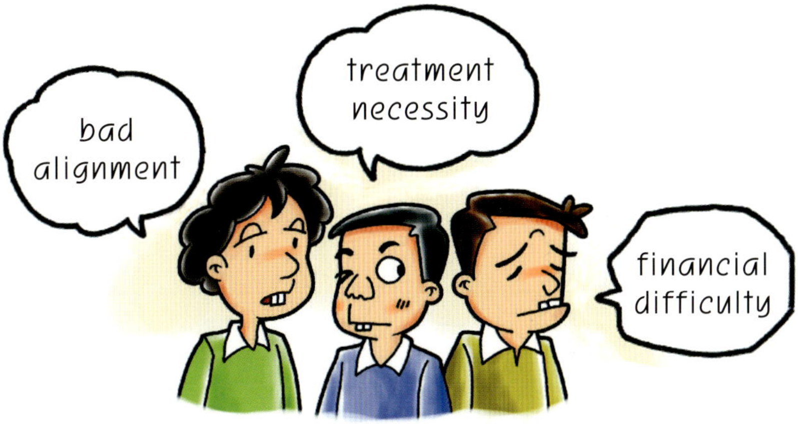

The practice and demand of orthodontic treatment differs among social classes and where they live. If the number of people who need treatments are similar between country and urban areas, it is more common for people who are living in cities can receive orthodontic treatments.

The demand for orthodontic treatment usually depends on family income, and social status also plays an important role in deciding orthodontic treatment. A person with higher social status and prestige will more likely desire to have better appearance.

Thus, people who are living in cities will be more likely to get orthodontic treatments.

7. Poorly Aligned Teeth Are Causes of the Following Discomforts

A. Obstacles for a Harmonious Social Life
B. Schematic View of Muscles around Head and Neck
C. Abnormal Curvature of Backbone(Spine)
D. Problems with Chewing
E. Normal Swallowing
F. Problems with Swallowing
G. Process of Swallowing Food
H. Mispronunciation while Speaking
I. Mispronunciation in the Early Ages.
J. Trauma to the Front Tooth.
K. Cavities
L. Why Difficulties in Thorough Brushing Exist?
M. Normal Structure of Periodontal Ligament
N. Favorable and Unfavorable Force Directions during Chewing
O. Gum Disease(Periodontitis)
P. Inefficient Jaw Developing
Q. Progressive Facial Changes from Cradle to Death
R. Changing Facial Shape and Subsequent Changes in Pronunciation

A. Obstacles for a Harmonious Social Life

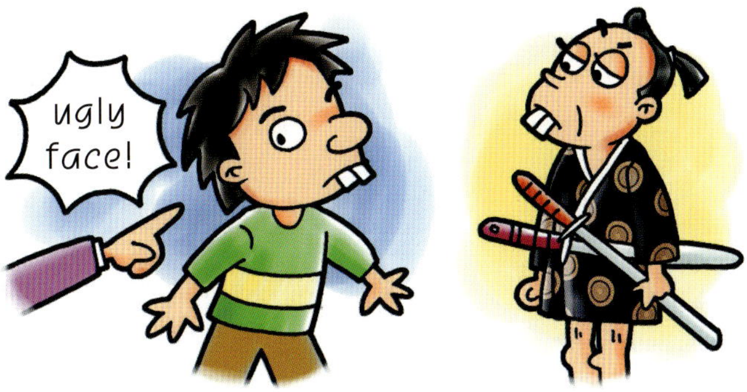

Having an interest in one's facial appearance can affect one's life style. People with a protruded upper jaw, or highly positioned upper canine can be ridiculed by others with nicknames such as "Bucktooth", "Witch Granny", or "Dracula".

In Western countries, a characteristic of having a protruded upper jaw plays a stereotypical role of underachieving individuals. So cartoonists often draw a character with protruding front teeth in order to depict a stupid person. Likewise, some cartoonists draw a Japanese character with protruded upper front teeth wearing a geta (Japanese sandal) and a hundoshi (Japanese loincloth).

In any society, a smile with neatly aligned teeth is considered to be beautiful, while poorly aligned teeth are thought to be unattractive.

Being attractive may play a considerable role in getting a job and choosing a spouse. If someone experiences an unpleasant incident due to his/her poorly aligned teeth, it is a serious problem that cannot be ignored.

B. Schematic View of Muscles around Head and Neck.

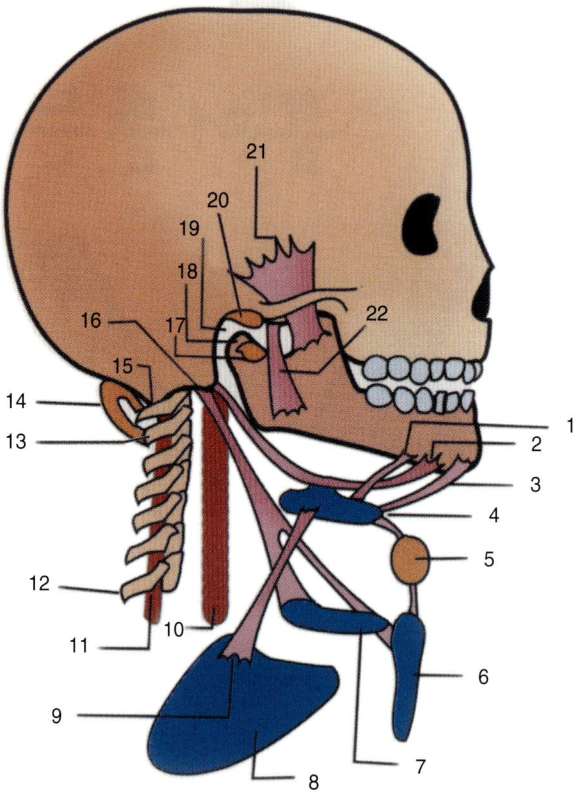

1. mylohyoid m.	12. 7th cervix
2. digastric m.	13. 2nd cervix
3. geniohyoid m.	14. occipital m.
4. hyoid bone	15. 1st. cervix
5. thyroid gland	16. sternomastoid m.
6. sternum	17. external pterygoid m.
7. clavicle	18. condylar process
8. scapula	19. temporomandibular joint
9. omohyoid m.	20. internal pterygoid m.
10. carotid artery	21. temporal m.
11. vertebral artery	22. masseter m

* "m." means muscle.

C. Abnormal Curvature of Backbone(Spine)

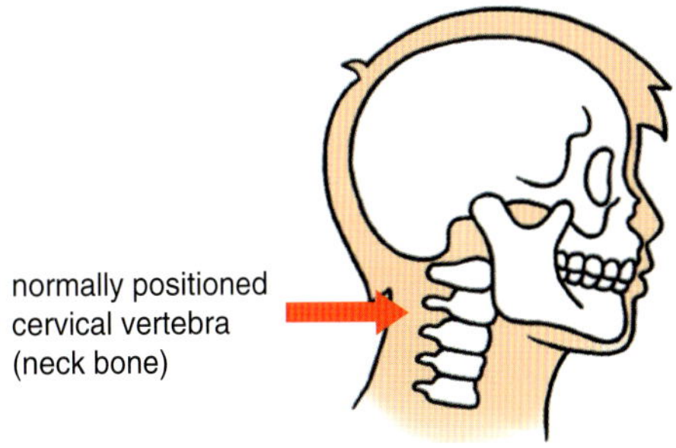

Because the relationship between the upper and lower teeth are normal, the structure of cervical vertebra(neck backbone) is arranged correctly.

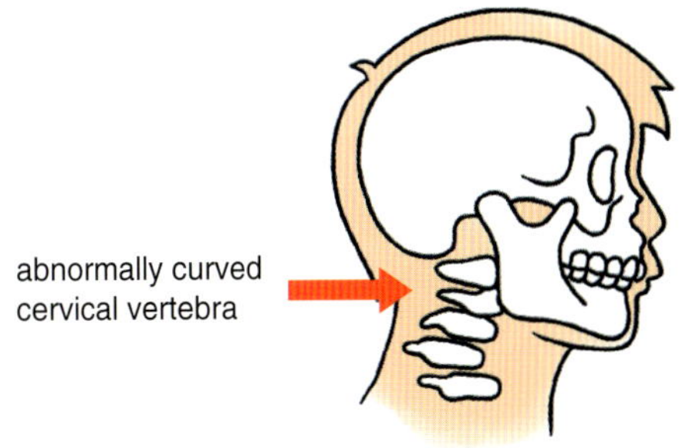

Because the relationship between the upper and lower teeth are abnormal, the cervical vertebra is being abnormally curved in this case.

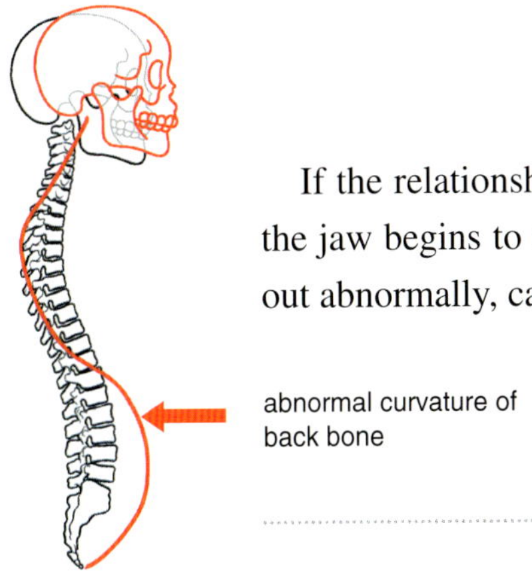

If the relationship between the upper and lower teeth are abnormal, the jaw begins to tilt outwards and the backbone starts to curve in and out abnormally, causing bad posture of the entire body.

D. Problems With Chewing

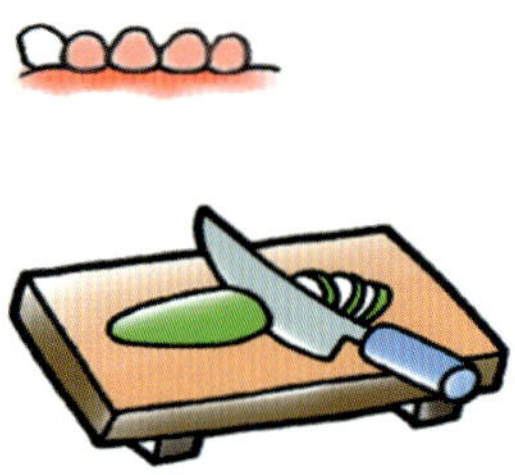

front teeth(cutting)

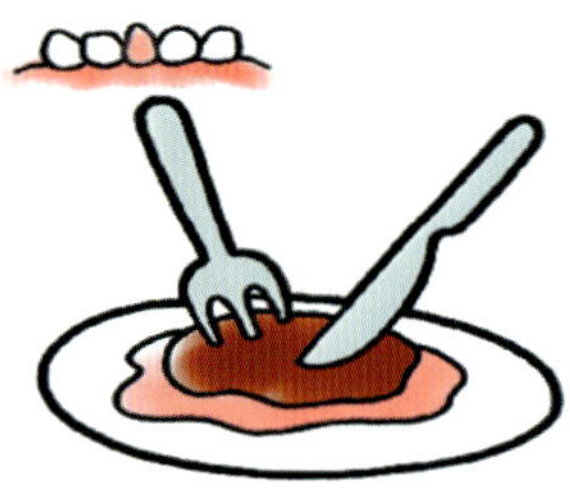

canine(tearing)

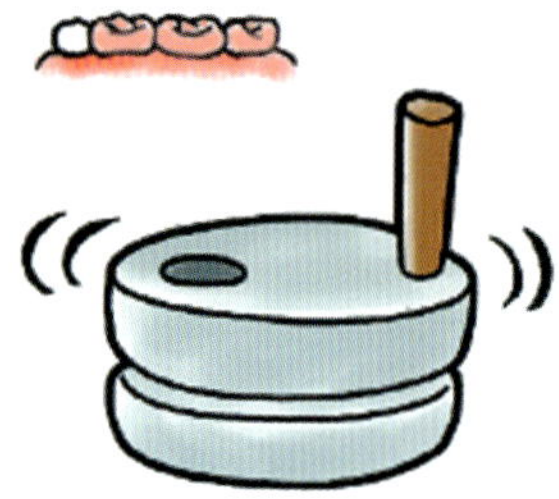

molar(crushing)

One of the most important functions of the teeth is chewing. To find out if your teeth are in good condition or not, try to chew tough cold Korean noodles named Naengmyon or Kimchi(a kind of Korean fermented vegetables).

People with a normal alignment of teeth will take in the food with their front teeth and lips, and tear with canine teeth. Next, the food is crushed with their molar teeth, then the chewed food mixed with saliva is swallowed down to the throat. Thus, chewing is considered to be the first step in getting the needed nutritions for the body.

Many adults who suffer from bad alignments of teeth get orthodontic treatments because they want to enjoy eating delicious foods such as cold noodles, Kimchi and Kalbi (grilled ribs). Basically, these are the foods that they can not eat properly if they have bad alignment of the front teeth.

I have treated many of these types of patients, and they are very satisfied with the results of chewing their food after orthodontic treatment. Some patients say they felt chewing sensation for the first time just after orthodontic treatments.

E. Normal Swallowing

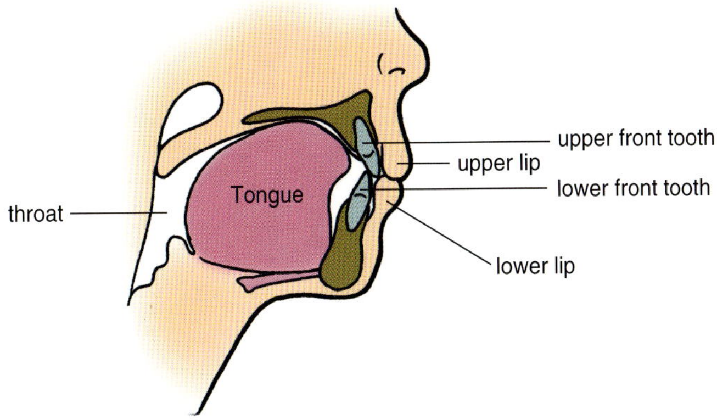

In case of normal swallowing, all teeth are in contact, upper and lower lips are closed, the upper surface of the tongue is elevated to touch the roof of mouth.

F. Abnormal Swallowing

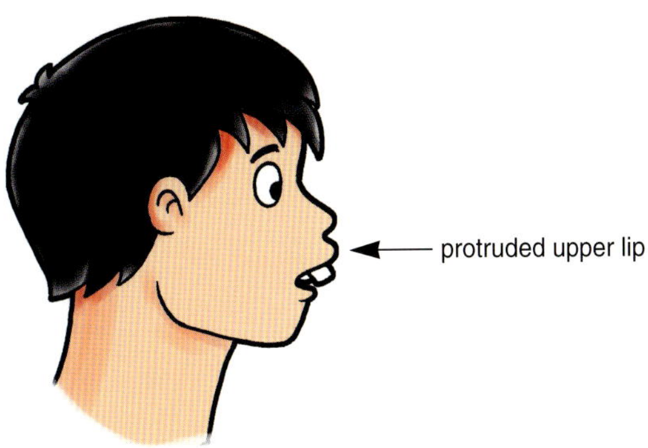

People with protruded upper jaw or long and tilted lower jaw have difficulties in swallowing. For most people who have normally aligned teeth, swallowing saliva does not involve any tension around the mouth. However, even if there is a horizontal gap of 2~3mm between the upper and lower front teeth, it would be very difficult to swallow saliva.

If the upper jaw is protruded and teeth are held apart during swallowing, the lips must be closed with a force or the lower lip must touch the inner side of the front teeth of the upper jaw to keep the tongue in the oral cavity and to seal. Thus swallowing can be completed. There is necessarily a strong activities of muscles around the lips to help swallowing.

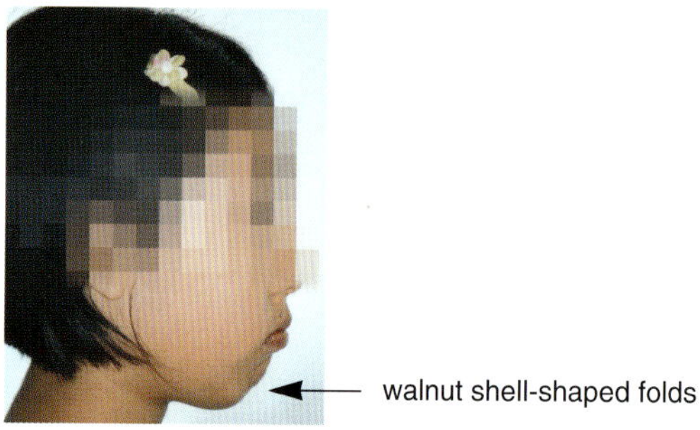

This will result in dimples on each side of the cheeks and create uneven walnut shell-shaped folds are formed on the lower region of the lower lip.

And if you repeat swallowing saliva in this condition, muscles around the lips and neck get extremely tired. Therefore, people with protruded upper jaw, long and tilted lower jaw, gap in-between their teeth(openbite) will have to live with unnecessary troubles for years, while others do not.

G. Process of Swallowing Food

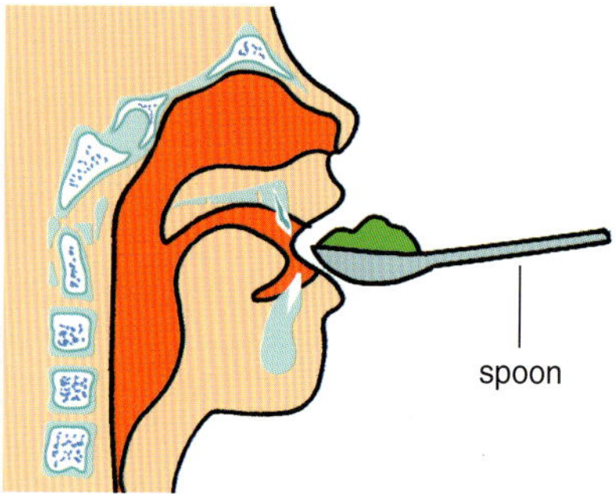

1. Food is inserted into the mouth with a spoon.

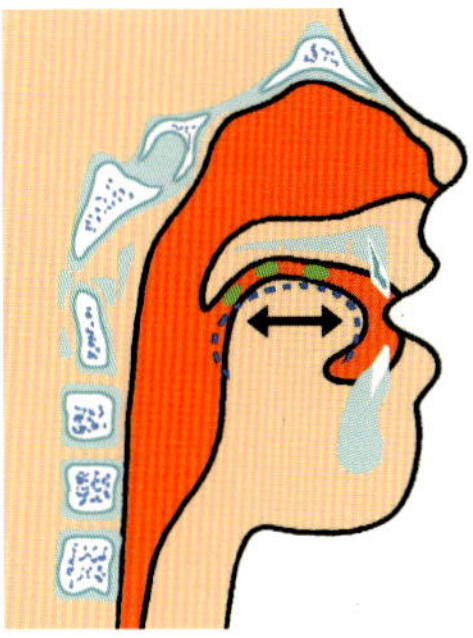

2. Even with soft foods, you must chew at least 10 times. For hard foods, you have to chew at least 30~50 times.

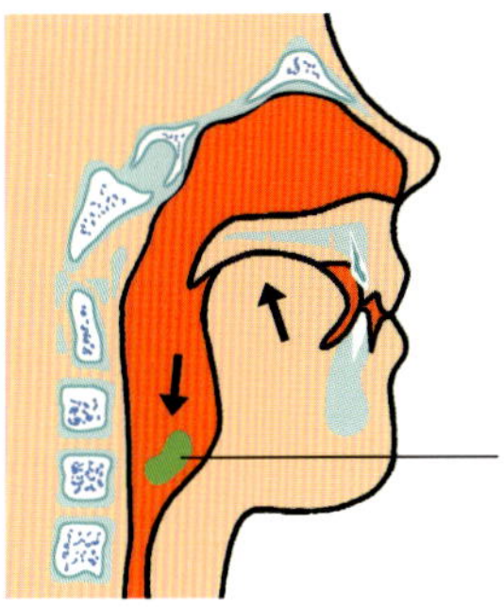

3. While being chewed, the food gets mixed with saliva. And with the aid of the tongue, the food moves down to the throat.

H. Mispronunciation while Speaking

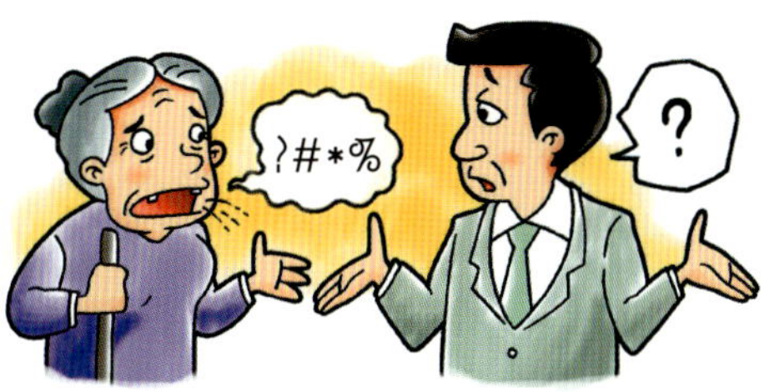

Since we think that we can pronounce words only with our tongue and lips, we are apt to think that speaking is possible even without teeth. However, the absence of teeth would make it impossible to pronounce words accurately, and also make your face wrinkled. This can often be seen with elderly persons, who speak with no teeth. Even with one missing front tooth, it is difficult to pronounce words accurately because of a whistling sound that results.

I. Mispronunciation in the Early Ages.

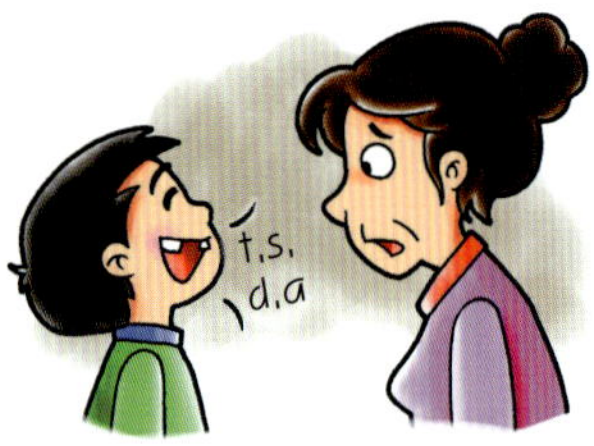

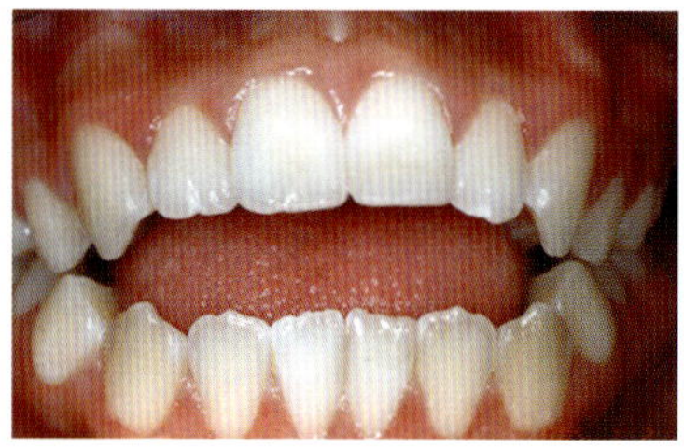

If you examine children who have the condition where the front teeth of upper and lower jaws are not contact due to the habit of sucking fingers for a long time, you will see that their pronunciation is incoherent compared to other kids of their ages, and spitting occurs while speaking. Because speaking is an essential part of social life, it is very important to learn how to pronounce words correctly from an early ages.

J. Trauma to the Front Teeth

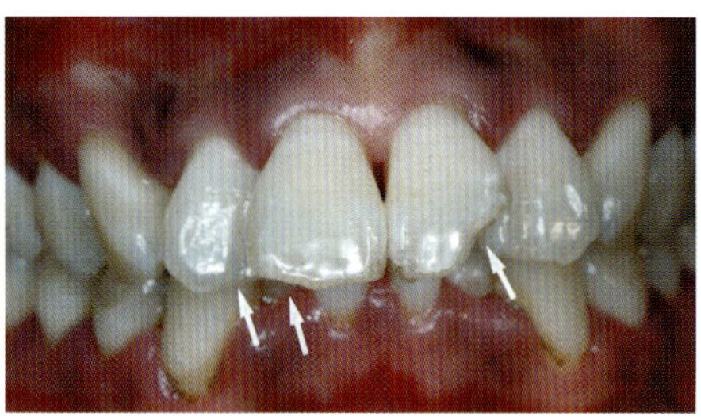

This patient is undergoing treatment because his front teeth of the upper jaw were fractured due to an external trauma to the mouth.

People with a protruded upper front teeth have a higher chance of fracturing those teeth during physical activities.

One out of every four children who have protruded upper teeth have experienced fracturing their front teeth during physical activities such as football game, rugby, judo, ice hockey, and taekwondo. One of the reasons why people treat protruded teeth at an early age is to lower the possibilities of this unexpected accident.

K. Cavities

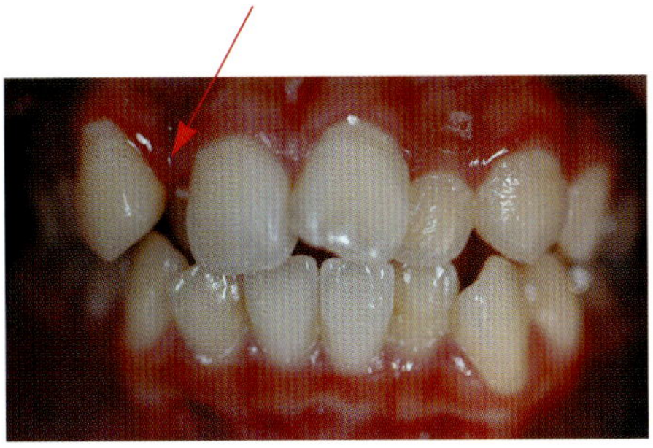
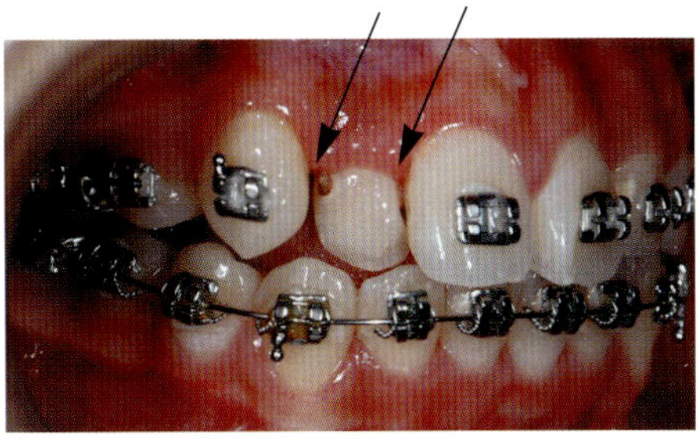

There are areas that have not been brushed properly. Even though many cavities are already existed before treatment, but remain unseen because of clustered teeth arrangement. As the teeth become neatly aligned after treatment, cavities become revealed.

Many people believe that teeth that are somewhat clustered together will not result in problems while eating food, and only through tooth brushing will lead to a good oral health in the years to come. But in reality, crowded teeth have areas where the tooth brush cannot reach.

Some patients visit me to get orthodontic treatments because of crowded teeth alignment, and they find out and think those cavities are increased with treatment.

But the truth is that cavities were present even before treatment began. As the teeth were beginning to align themselves properly, the cavities naturally became revealed.

If teeth are poorly aligned, it is recommended to receive orthodontic treatments as soon as possible. This way, cavities can be prevented.

L. Why Difficulties in Thorough Brushing Exist?

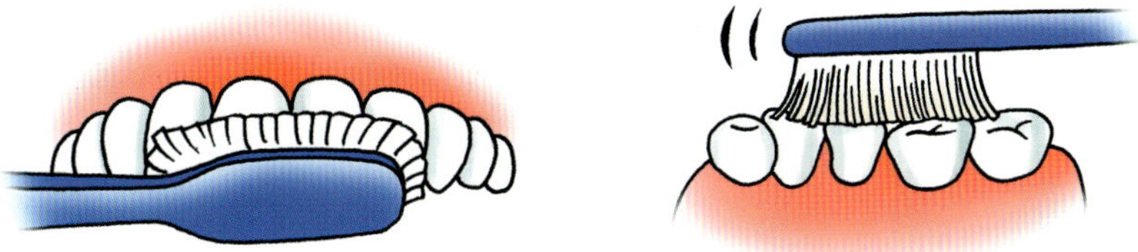

If the teeth are aligned properly, brushing is easy.

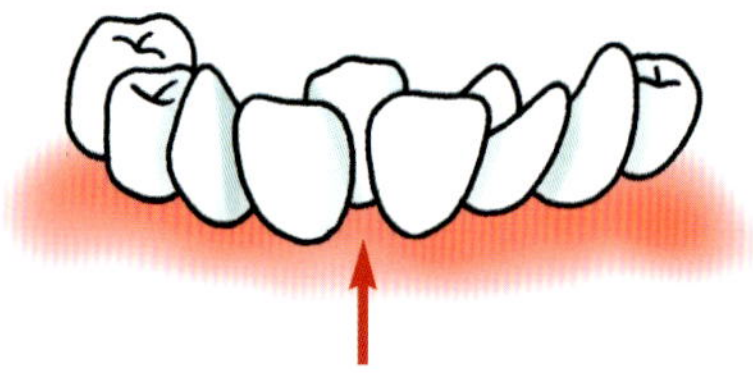

Clustered teeth, viewed from the front.
Tooth brush cannot reach arrow area.

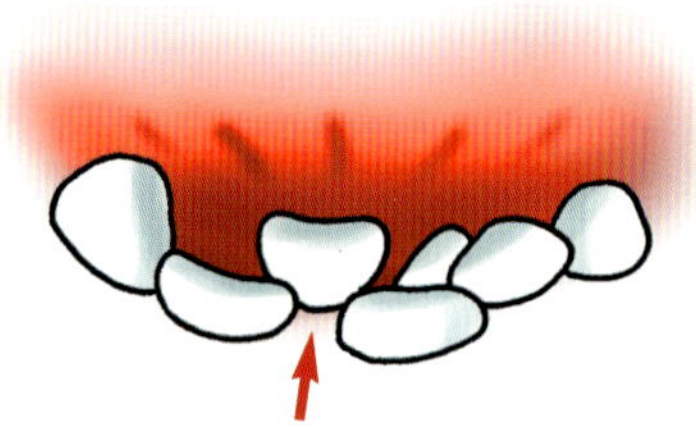

Viewed from the top.

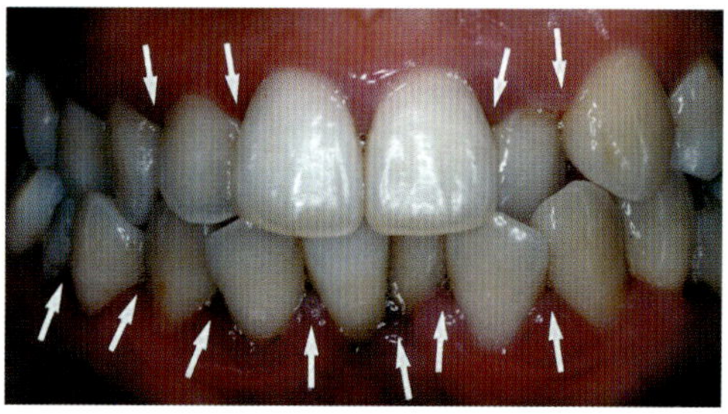

Severe gum disease(periodontitis) and heavily deposited dental calculus are recognized because of lacking in tooth brushing.

The toothbrush should reach in between the teeth to maintain cleanliness, but this is quite difficult if the teeth are clustered. Therefore, a good alignment of teeth by orthodontic treatments is necessary in order to make it easier to brush the teeth.

M. Normal Structure of Periodontal Ligament

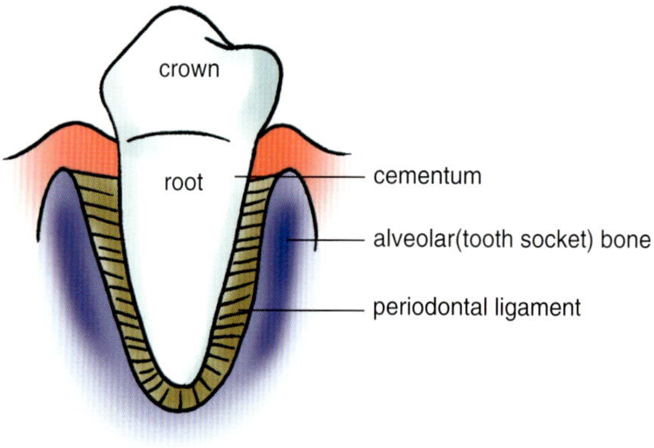

Periodontal ligament is present between the root of the tooth and the alveolar(tooth socket) bone which lines the tooth socket. It is composed of collagenous connective fibers that suspend the tooth in the bony socket. Most of these fibers run obliquely from the surface of the root called cementum, extending upward (occlusally) to attach in the alveolar bone.

Since the teeth are constantly receiving biting forces and when the force is applied to the tooth, periodontal ligament act as a natural shock absorber.

N. Favorable and Unfavorable Force Directions during Chewing

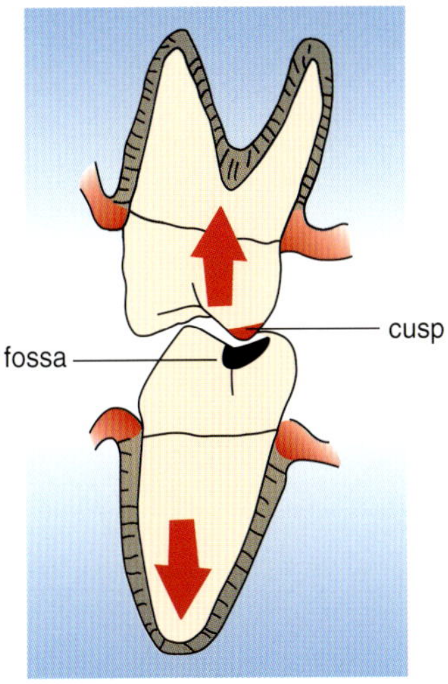

Favorable Force Direction

When cusp tips contact the fossa area of the opposing tooth, the resultant force is directed vertically through the long axis of the tooth (arrow). This type of force is favorable for the health of periodontal ligament.

If the teeth alignment between upper and lower jaw is in good condition, biting forces during chewing are directed vertically through the long axis of the teeth. This type of force is favorable for health of the tooth.

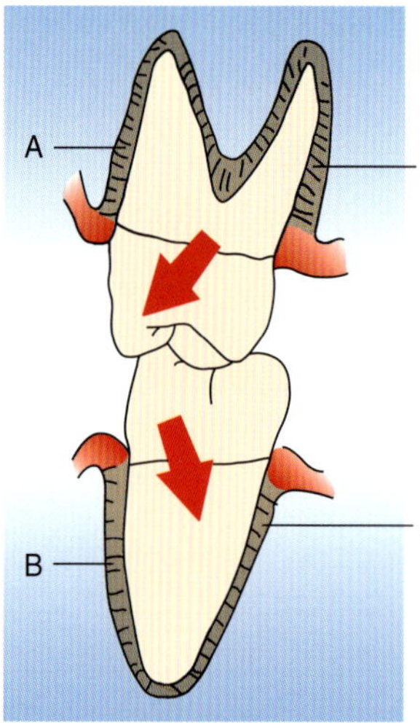

Direction of force is not through the long axis of the teeth. Resultant tipping forces are created (arrows) that tend to cause compression(A) of certain areas of periodontal ligament and elongation (B) of other areas.

Unfavorable Force Direction

When a tooth is contacted on an inclined plane, the resultant force is not directed through its long axis which is unfavorable for the health of teeth. In this case, unfavorable tipping forces are created, resulting in destruction of the alveolar bone.

O. Gum Disease(Periodontitis)

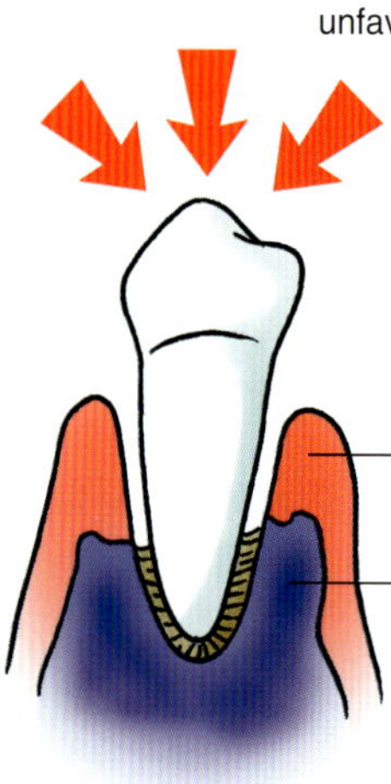

Damaged alveolar bone caused by over pressure applied to a bad positioned tooth.

With poorly aligned dentition, there are teeth that are in good contact with opposing teeth, but there are also teeth that are out of contact or heavily contacted.

Regarding the teeth that are out of contact, there is not enough stimulation during chewing, and this results in poor blood circulation around the individual tooth.

With teeth that are heavily contacted, there can be too much pressure. If too much pressure is applied to only one or two teeth, the periodontal ligament cannot absorb the biting forces. This leads to damaging the alveolar bone of relevant teeth and this causes the tooth to be loosened.

This causes an imbalance in the structural functions of the teeth, and these are the main causes of weakening the overall health of the teeth.

P. Inefficient Jaw Developing

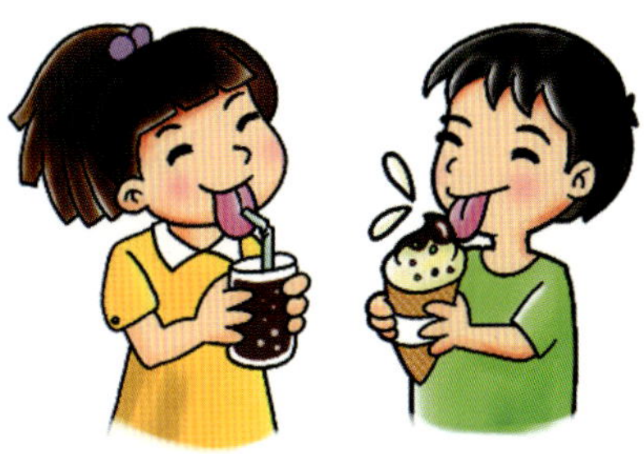

If the teeth of upper and lower jaws are in good conditions with each other, the jaws will be able to develop normally. Compared to primitive ancestors who ate tough meats, hard beans and nuts, and fruits, modern people eat soft refined foods. This led us to have smaller jaws, and at the same time, our jaw muscles were not used enough, as a consequence, the jaw itself has become weaker.

Properly aligned teeth that can break down hard food materials are very important factor for growing children. Fast foods are not only bad for their general health, but also may deteriorate the effective development of their jaws.

Q. Progressive Facial Change from Cradle to Death

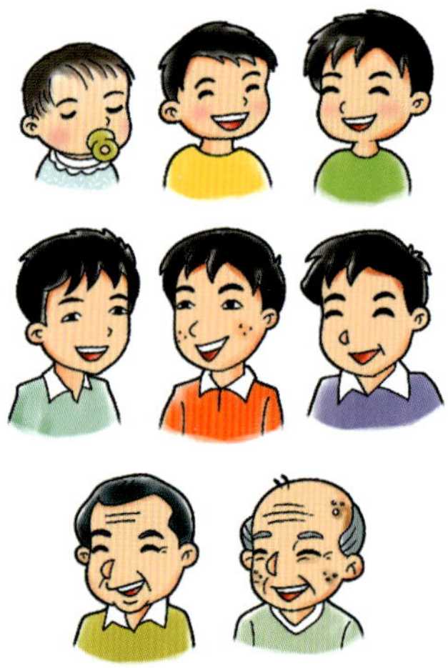

If they have their natural teeth, they look young and very healthy.

R. Changing Facial Shape and Subsequent Changes in Pronunciation

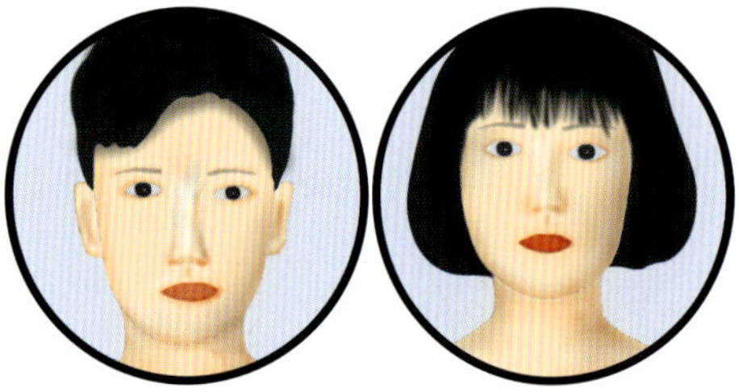

past beauty

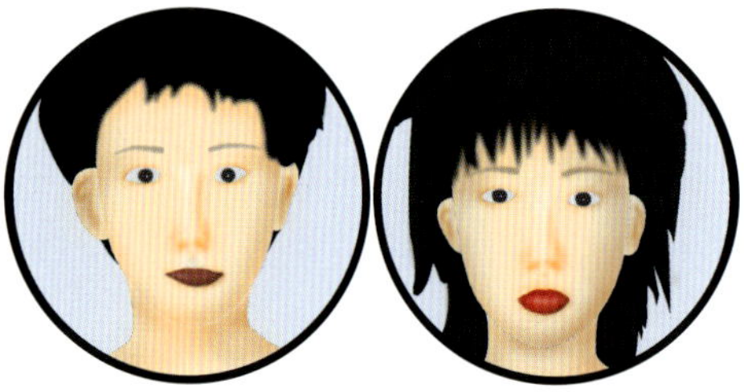

modern beauty

As modernization has progressed, the use of the muscles around the head and neck regions has become less frequent. It leads to a smaller distance between the eyes and cheekbones, and smaller jaws. Noses became higher and the face width became narrower. According to the recent studies, the pronunciation of Korean language is changing because of small-sized jaw. These facts prove that the proper development of the jaws depends on the dietary habit.

8. Neatly Aligned Teeth Give You Following Blessings.

A. Good Memory

B. Good Blood Circulations to the Brain.

C. Better Motor Skills of the Body

D. Strong Body Structure

E. Stimulation of Lymphatic Vessels

F. Prevention of Weakening the Eyesight

G. Prevention of Overweight

H. Positive Attitude Toward Life

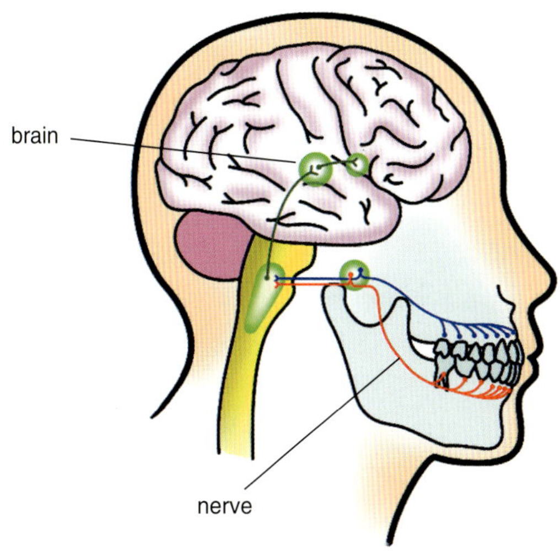

A. Good Memory

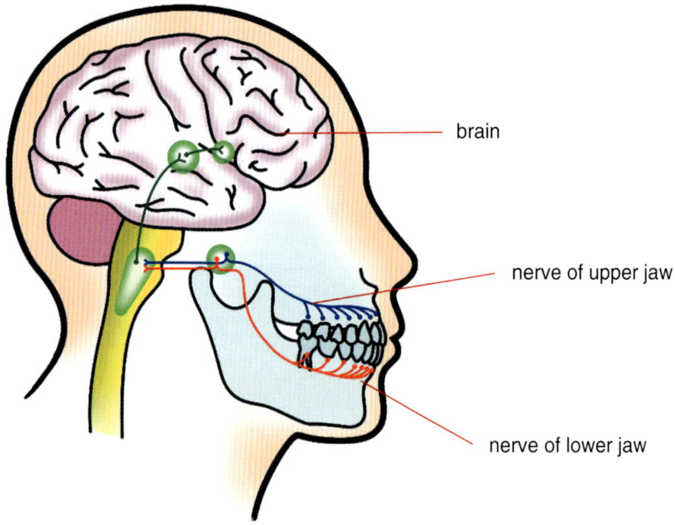

Chewing stimulates to increase blood circulation to the brain. Thus, when someone becomes drowsy while driving, chewing gum is much more effective than drinking coffee or caffeine containing tea. By chewing gums, blood circulation to the brain increases, so its functions become more active. To develop children's intellect and to prevent dementia of the senior citizens, it is important for the brain to be active.

In the case of the elderly who can chew food effectively, a large amount of blood circulates to the brain. The pressure applied to the teeth while chewing food also will stimulate the brain through the periodontal ligament of the teeth. As a result, this could cause the slower aging process of the brain.

B. Good Blood Circulations to the Brain

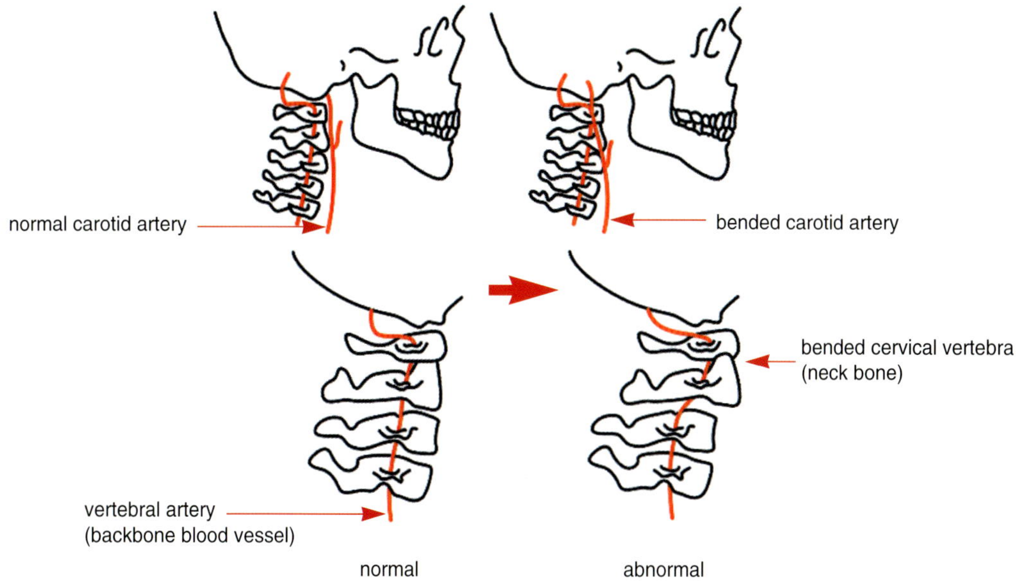

The carotid and vertebral artery to brain pass through cervical vertebra region. With properly aligned teeth, the position of the cervical vertebra is in place and there is no disturbance to the blood circulation. This leads to positive functioning of the brain.

If the relationship between the upper and lower teeth is abnormal, the cervical vertebra bends in the direction of the arrow. Then, the carotid and vertebral arteries are bended, causing a disturbance of blood circulation to the brain. With poor blood circulation to brain, the functions of the brain become less effective.

Growing children with poorly aligned teeth cannot chew well. This leads to less stimulation to the brain, having a negative effect on the child's development of intelligence.

Even for the elderly, chewing is very important because it is much more effective means for the stimulation of the brain. The biting forces applied to the teeth while chewing is transmitted to the brain via periodontal ligament, leading to activate the brain function.

C. Better Motor Skills of the Body

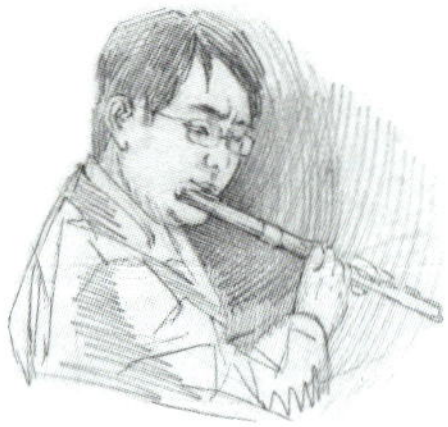
general person 100

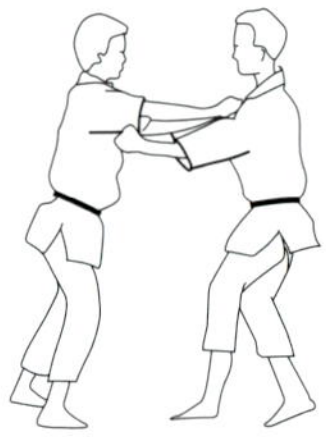
judo player 146

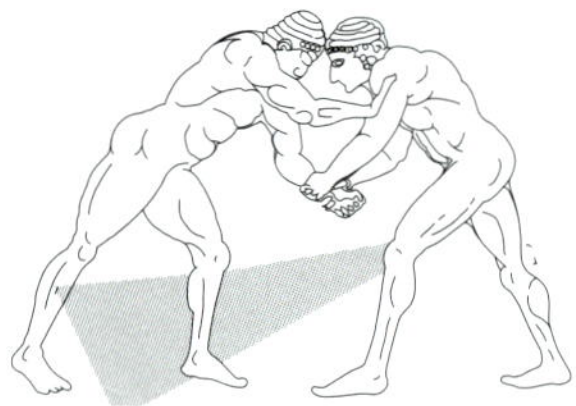
wrestler 158

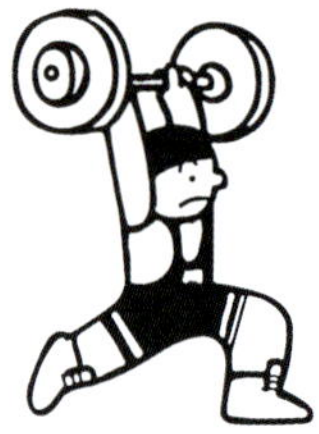
weight lifter 208

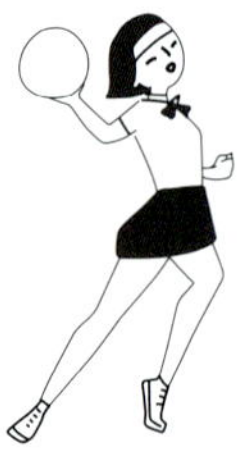
handball player 210

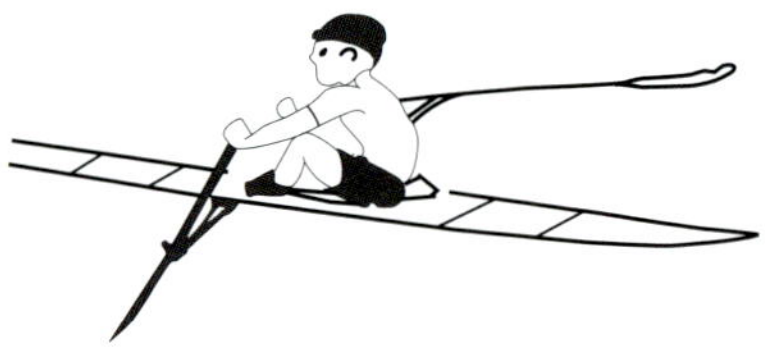
rower 288

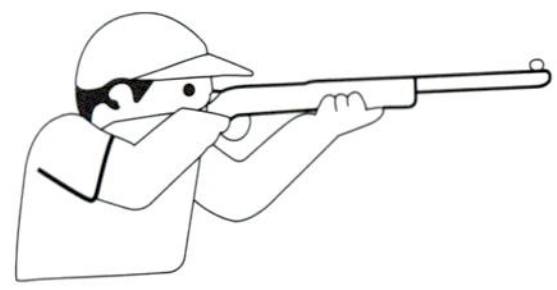
shooter 295

Comparison of Biting Forces

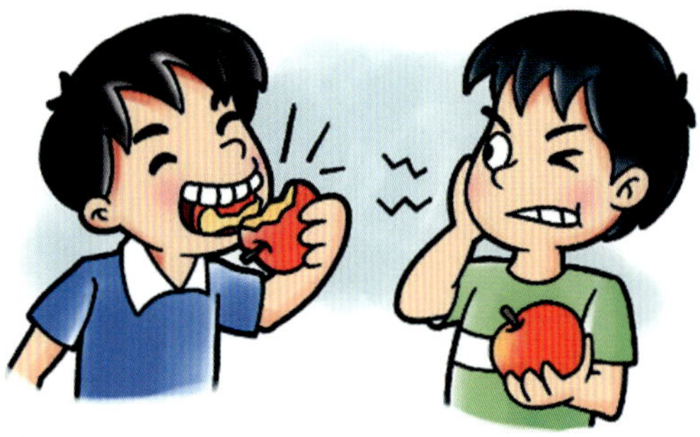

Generally, children who chew well have superior levels of strength, thus they can run faster or throw farther than other kids. In addition, chewing force is correlated to the development of abdominal muscles, increased grasping power, and other types of motor skills. You may notice that most athletes have neatly aligned teeth.

D. Strong Body Structure

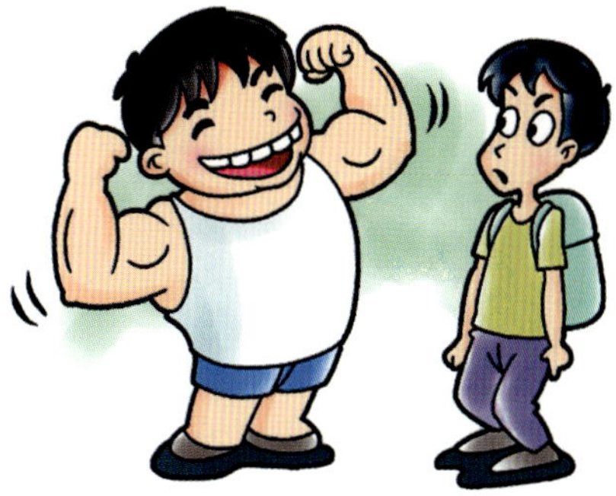

It is a well-known fact that the more you chew, the more saliva is excreted. Saliva contains a substance called parotin. It stimulates digestion and helps strengthen the teeth, bones, muscles, and blood vessels. Saliva also serves as self-cleansing the oral cavity.

E. Stimulation of Lymphatic Vessels

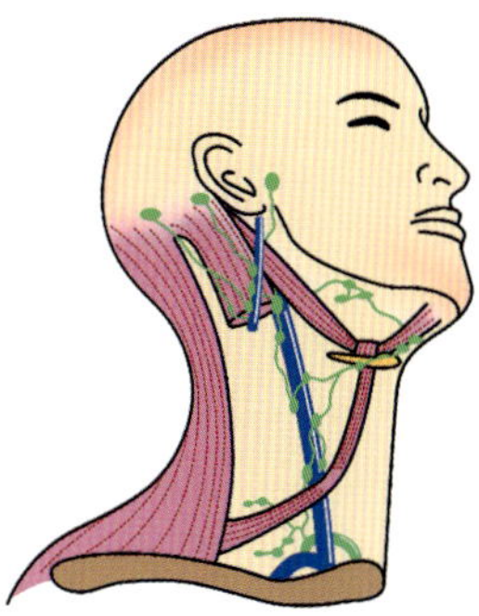

Green color indicates lymph nodes. Many lymph nodes are located near the neck

Chewing for an extended period of time stimulates the lymphatic vessels within the head and neck region, making a healthier body. One-third of the lymph nodes in the body is located near the head and neck.

F. Prevention of Weakening the Eyesight

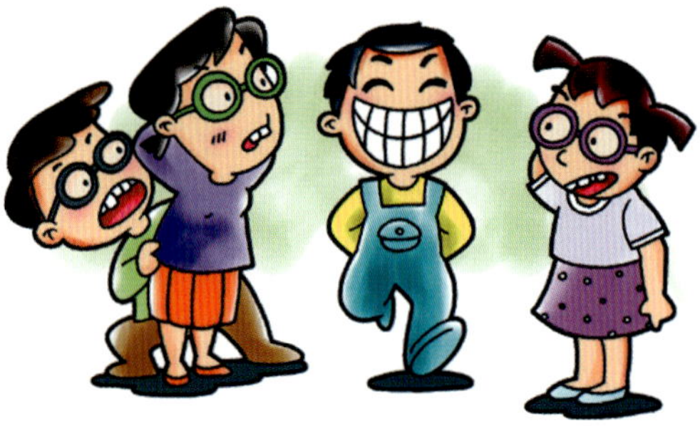

These days, weakening of the eyesight among children has increased tremendously. It is commonly concluded that television, cartoons and video games are the main factors for such a phenomenon.

However, recent studies indicate that the main reason for weakening the eyesight may be attributed to control difficulties of crystalline lens of the eyes caused by lowered function of facial muscles. A good habit of chewing food properly could protect eyesight by increasing the strength of facial muscles.

G. Prevention of Overweight

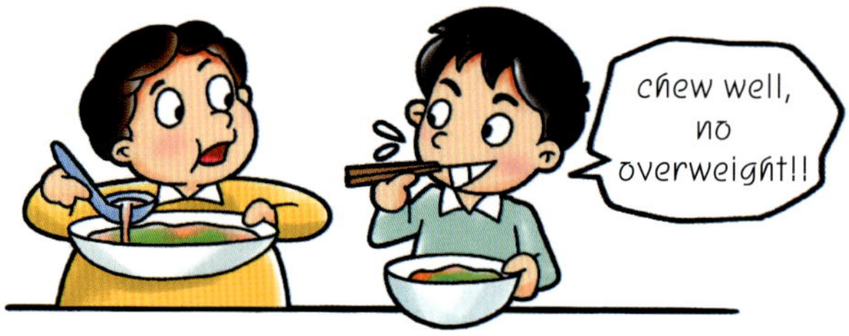

Lower chewing frequency leads to overweight

Higher chewing frequency increases the amount of excretion of saliva, which increases the rate of digestion process. Digestion of food will increase the level of blood sugar, that stimulates the brain's satire center. As a result, one's appetite decreases and then it causes to stop eating.

Lower chewing frequency lowers the level of the digestion, so the stimulation of the satire center occurs only after a considerable amount of food has been ingested, which could lead to overweight.

H. Positive Attitude toward Life

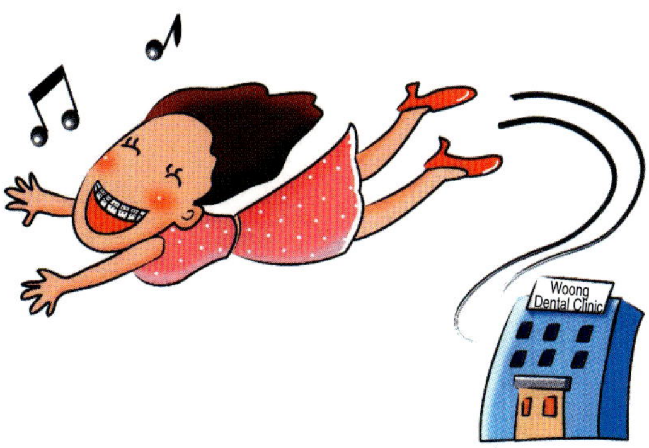

Many patients admit that their attitudes toward life have greatly changed after finishing orthodontic treatments. Some patients revealed that they were even afraid to take pictures or to simply talk to other people before the treatment. However, orthodontic treatment naturally removed this barrier and enabled them to socialize comfortably by talking and laughing with others. As a result, orthodontic treatment changed the patient's attitudes toward life.

Many patients also admit that after the orthodontic treatments, seeing their beautiful smile with perfectly aligned teeth made them even more happier than the fact that they can chew more comfortably and naturally.

A comment as follows from many patients who received orthodontic treatment brought great pride to me as an orthodontist;

"I feel like I am a totally new person now. Everyone says that my smile becomes very natural and they believe that it reflects how happy I am. Before the treatment, I wasn't even able to open my mouth in front of the others. But now, my life is filled with joy. If anyone is experiencing the same trouble as I did in the past, I would strongly recommend them to receive treatment from Dr. Lew. "

III. Breast Feeding and Nursing Bottle

9. Correlation between Feeding and Tooth Alignment

A. Breast Feeding

B. Swallowing Procedure of Breast Feeding

C. Non-Physiologic Nursing Bottle

D. Physiologic Nursing Bottle

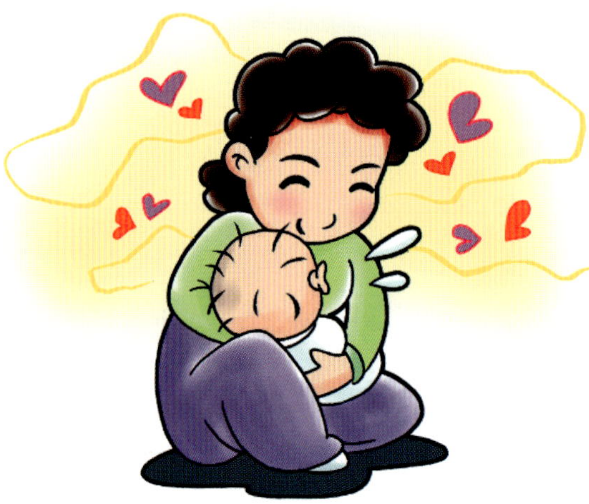

A. Breast Feeding

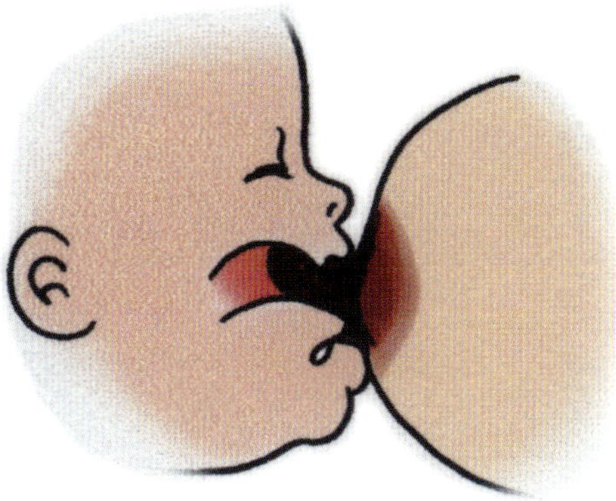

To raise a strong and healthy child, it is important to feed breast milk. Breast milk contains immunoglobulin and other enzymes that help the child to grow healthy.

The act of an infant suckling on mother's nipple will have different effects compared to a baby sucking on a bottle.

During the sucking period, the infant is developing its jaw, face, and neck muscles. The muscles surrounding the neck are connected to the entire body, so the muscle exercises play an important role in straightening the backbones.

For these reasons, babies raised with powdered milk may lack the development of the jaw bone, and this can lead to ineffective chewing and bad posture afterwards.

B. Swallowing Procedure of Breast Feeding

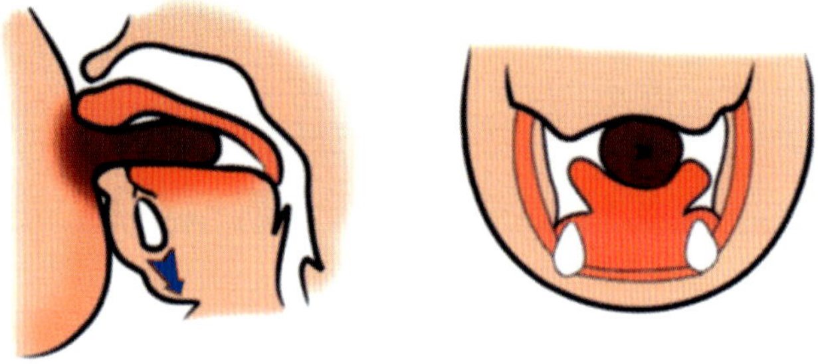

The infant lowers its lower jaw for opening the mouth.

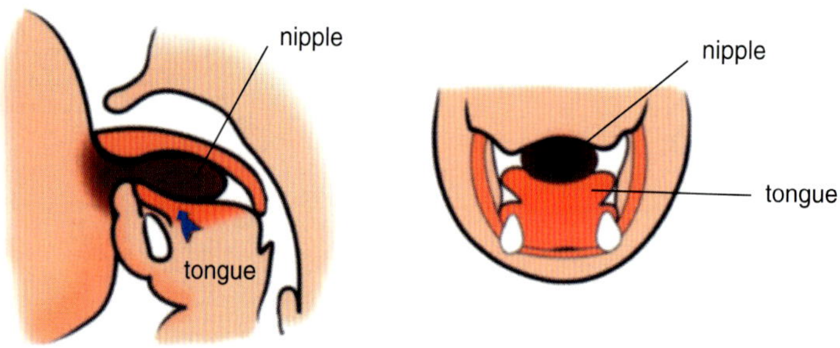

At the same time the tongue is placed anteriorly in contact with the lower lip, and squeezes out the milk in the breast.

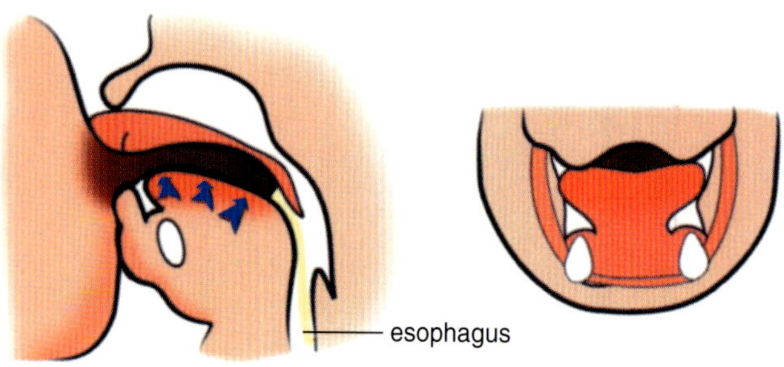

Breast milk is deposited on the tongue, and then groove the tongue in order to allow the milk to flow into the esophagus.

C. Non-Physiologic Nursing Bottle.

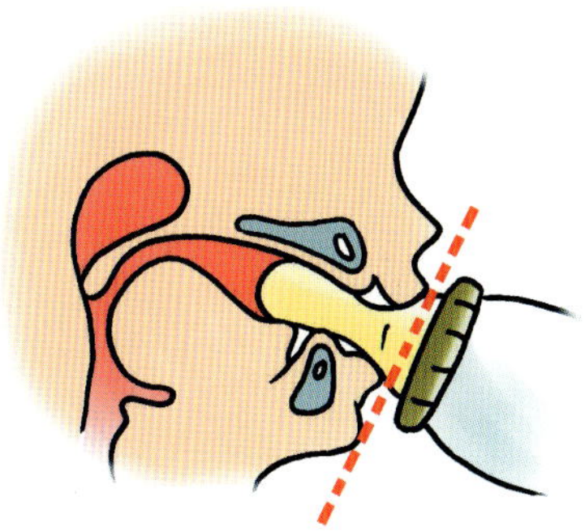

The mouth is opened unduly and makes a lip seal to be difficult. As a compensatory response to the unduly excessive opening movement required for non-physiologic nursing bottle, abnormal muscle pressures are exerted during sucking milk bottle. Also air intake during sucking is likely to occur.

D. Physiologic Nursing Bottle

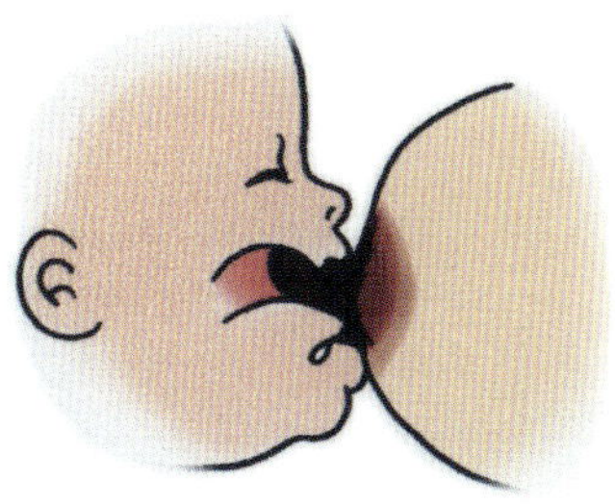

breast feeding

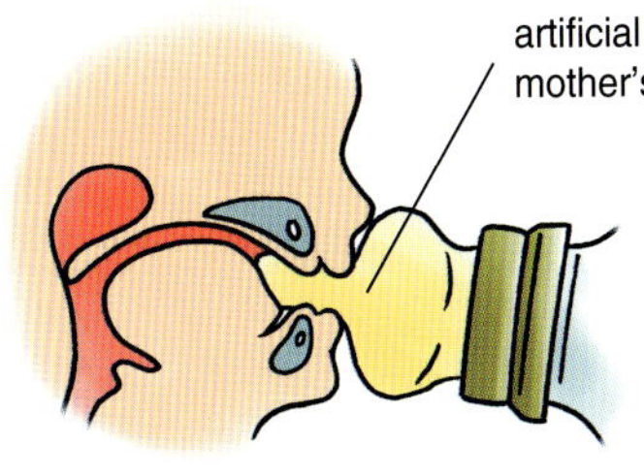

physiologic nursing bottle

Physiologic nursing bottle must closely resemble the natural activity of breast feeding. The entire area of upper and lower lips must be contacted the warm nipple base which is flexible and adapts to the contour of the baby lips. Although there are bottles that are almost identical to a mother's nipple, it cannot bring about exactly the same positive results as breast feeding.

IV. Occlusions

10. The Proper Setting of Teeth

A. Cusp and Fossa Relationship

B. Occlusion

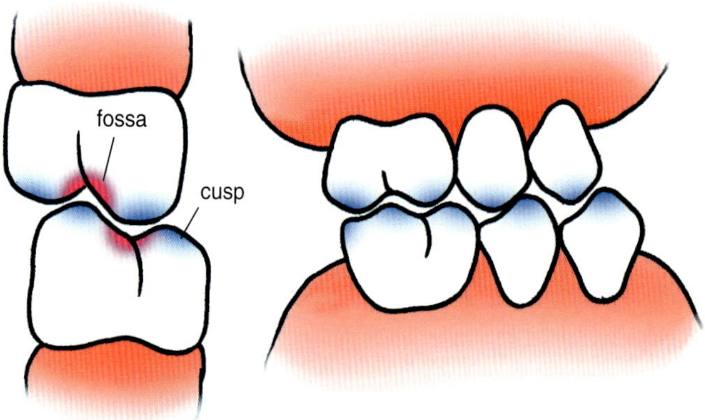

A. Cusp and Fossa Relationship

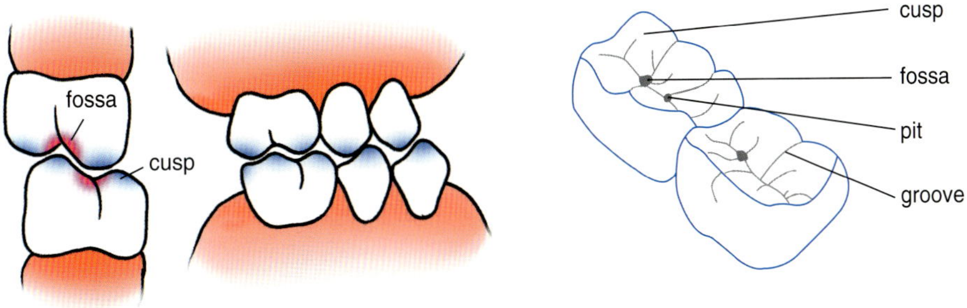

Blue zone is cusp, red zone is fossa and groove. Right illustration shows the surface of back teeth which come into contact with those of the opposite jaw during act of chewing, also called occlusal surface. Cusps, fossa, grooves, pits are shown.

Every tooth has several sets of little mountain top shapes called cusp. In between these tiny mountain tops lie little valleys called fossa and groove. Normally, when people's teeth begin to erupt, the upper and lower sets of cusp will structurally fit into the fossa and groove of the opposite jaws.

B. Occlusion

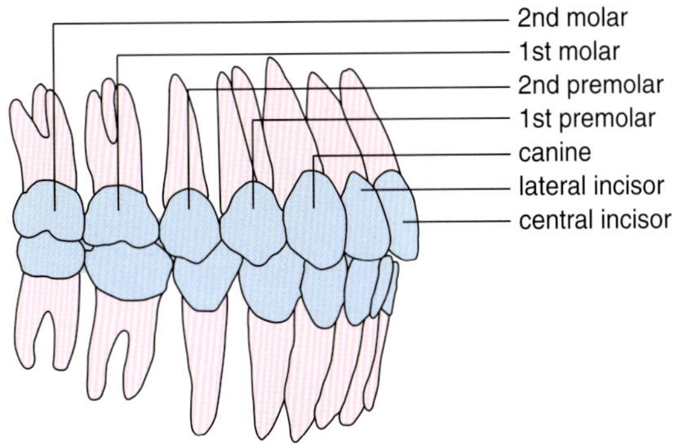

dentition and occlusion

The natural teeth in position in their alveolar(tooth) bone are referred to as dentition and the state of the teeth of the upper and lower jaw joining together is referred to as occlusion.

When the teeth of the upper and lower jaws are improperly joined together, it is called "malocclusion". Such malposition caused by abnormal contact of the upper and lower teeth interferes with normal oral functions such as chewing, pronunciation, and swallowing.

11. Classification of Malocclusion

A. Class I Malocclusion

B. Class II Malocclusion

C. Class III Malocclusion

A. Class I Malocclusion

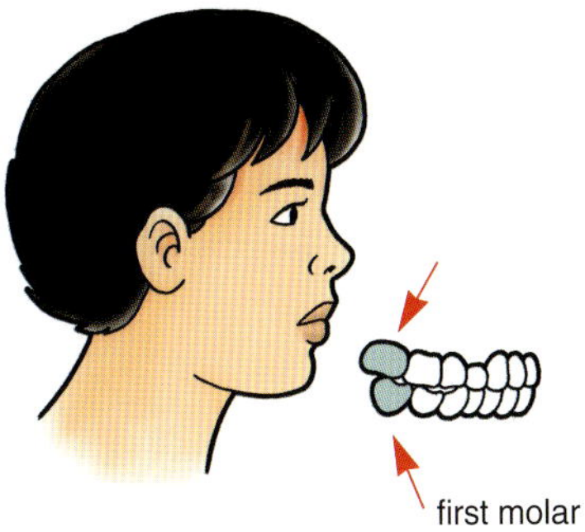

Class I malocclusion usually refers to an uneven set of teeth. It consists normal anterior-posterior relationship between upper and lower jaws, as indicated by correct fitting together of cusps and fossa of upper and lower first molars (blue-colored teeth), but crowding and rotation of teeth is happening elsewhere.

B. Class II Malocclusion

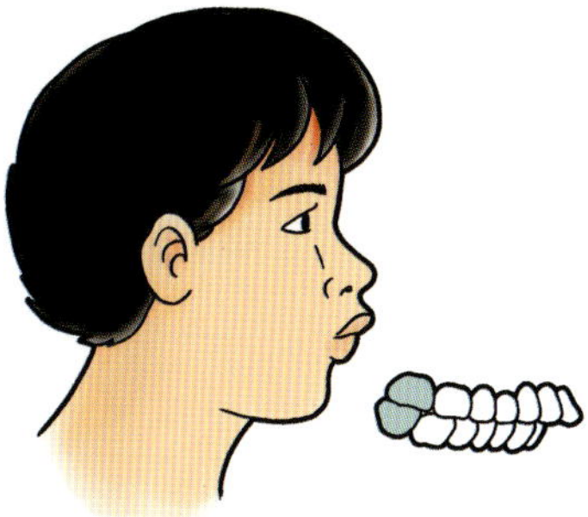

Class II malocclusion usually refers to protruded upper jaw. The lower jaw is posteriorly positioned to the upper one and the lower first molar is distal to the upper first molar.

C. Class III Malocclusion

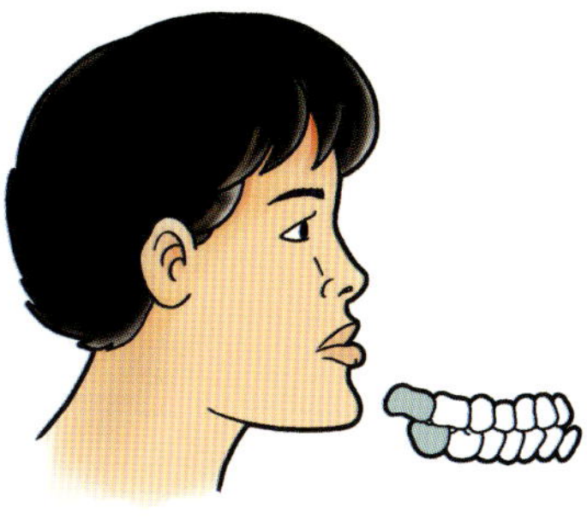

In case of Class III malocclusion, lower jaw is generally long and tilted downward. The lower jaw is anteriorly positioned to the upper one and the lower first molar is mesial to the upper first molar.

12. Circumstances Where Orthodontic Treatment Is Necessary.

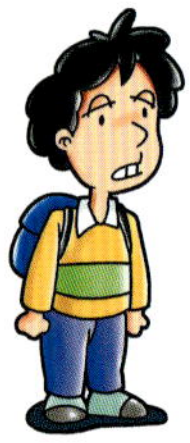
Teeth are always revealed.

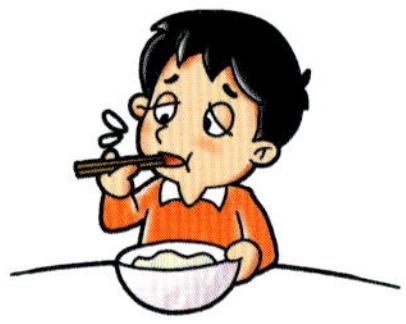
Chewing Food Roughly

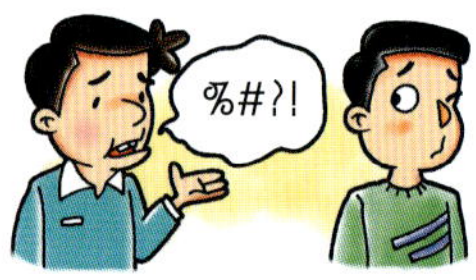

Incorrect Pronunciation

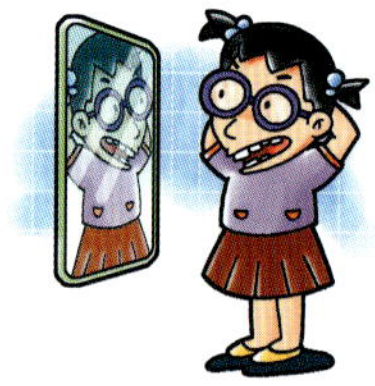
Concerned about Appearance

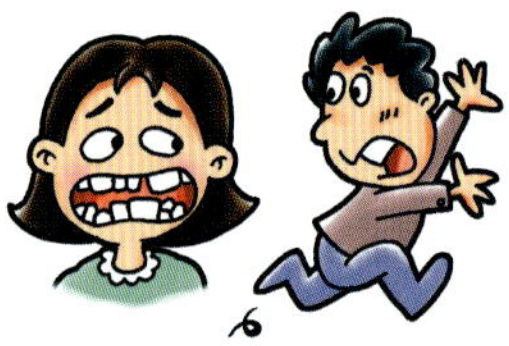
Poorly Aligned Teeth

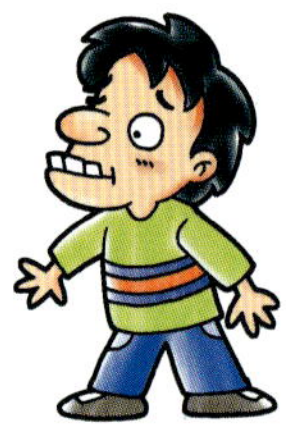
Long and Tilted downward Lower Jaw

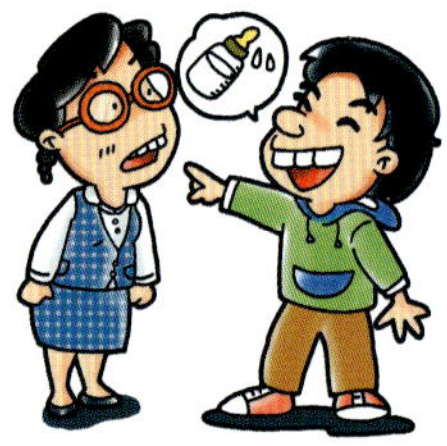
Milk Teeth Remained

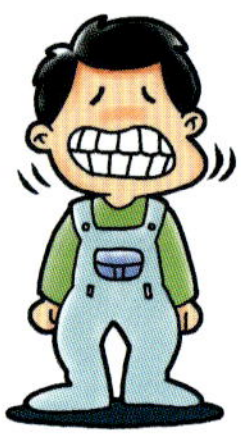
Asymmetric Face

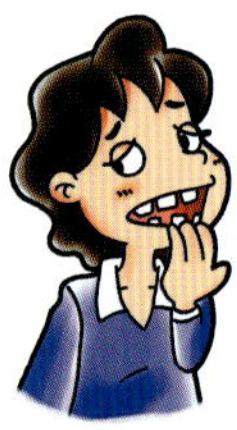
Sparsely Aligned Teeth

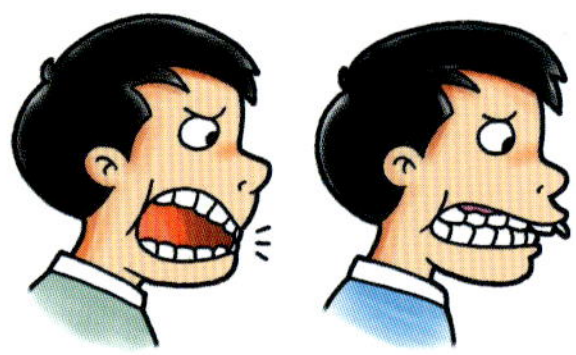
Gap between the Teeth of the Upper and Lower Jaw

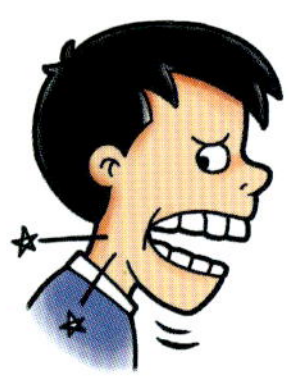
Clicking Sound of Jaw Joint during Chewing

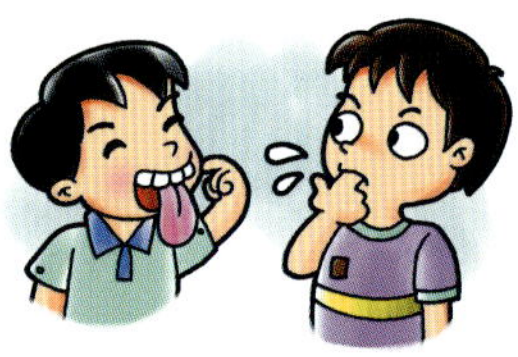
Thumb Sucking and/ or Tongue Thrusting

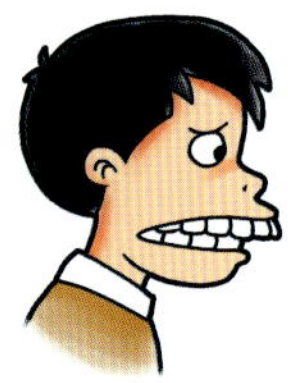
Protruded Upper Jaw

13. Best Time for Orthodontic Treatment

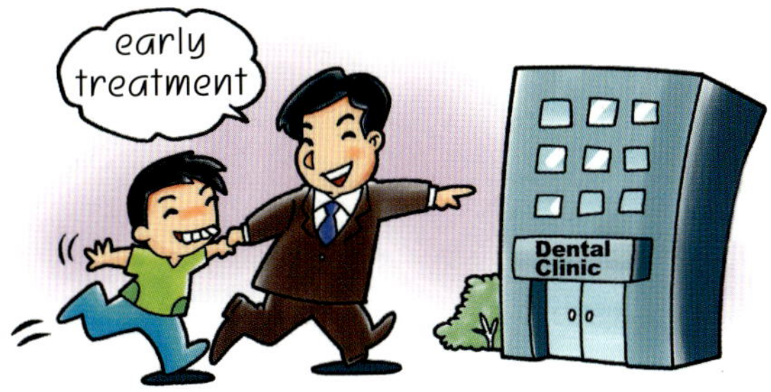

In general, around 12~14 years of age is good for orthodontic treatment.
In case of an adult patient, it takes longer for the teeth to move.

In general, around 12~14 years of age is good for orthodontic treatment. In case of an adult patient, it takes longer for the teeth to move.

The best time to start the treatment differs according to the conception of what is the best treatment for the patient. Therefore, it can be difficult to say when to start.

For people who think the shorter treatment period is the best, receiving treatment around 12~14 years of age just after all the permanent teeth eruption takes place might be a good time. At this time, the treatment will be finished in about 2 years.

However, we do not recommend a 7 to 8 year old patient to wait until 12~14 years of age just because of the short treatment period. It is the principle of orthodontic treatments to discover the problem early and to treat it in its early stages if possible.

V. Various Kinds of Malocclusions

14. Crowding

A. Slight Irregular Alignment of the Lower Front Teeth.

B. Definition of Leeway Space

C. Schematic View of Leeway Space

D. Improper Eruption Order Can Result in a Snag Canine

E. Discomfort Induced by Snag Canine

F. Even the Ancient Scholars Detested the Bad Alignment of the Teeth.

G. Could the Prime of Youth Cover the Handicap of Snag Canine Teeth?

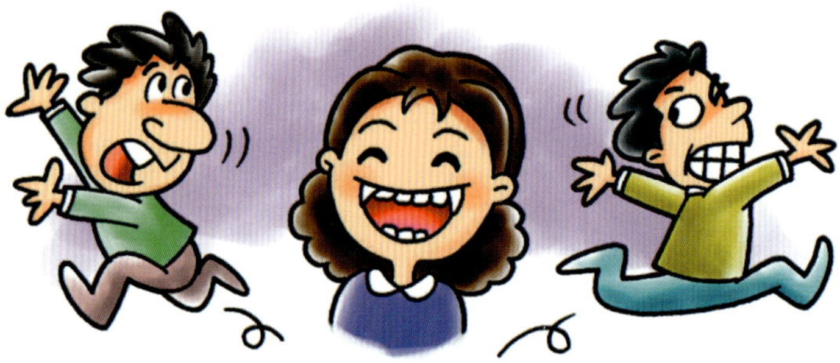

A. Slightly Irregular Alignment of the Lower Anterior Teeth

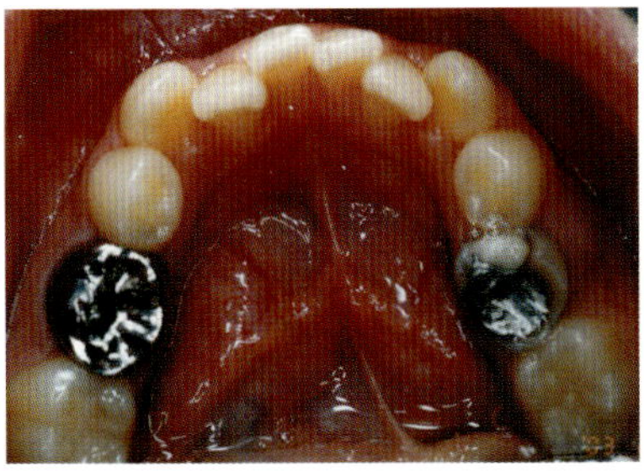

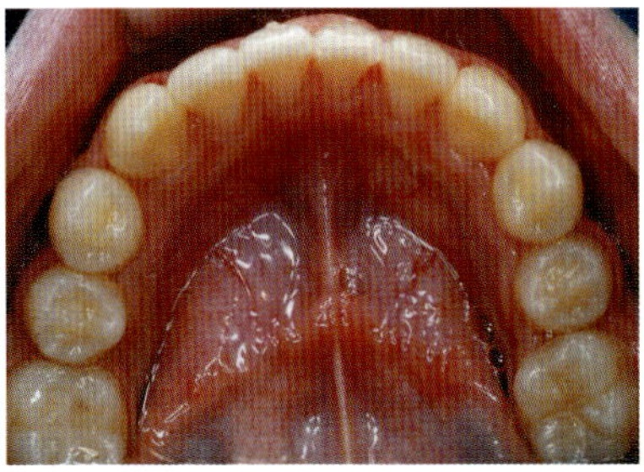

Improperly aligned, rotated, or snaggletooth are commonly referred to as crowding. Around the time a child enters elementary school, the adult front teeth of the lower jaw begin to erupt. At this stage, the teeth are aligned somewhat irregularly, but this type of teeth alignment is quite normal for children of this age and will disappear spontaneously without the aid of orthodontic treatments.

B. Definition of Leeway Space

The total width of the adult canine, first and second premolars erupting after the milk teeth shed, is smaller than those of deciduous(milk) canine, 1st, and 2nd molars, which leaves enough space for the proper alignment of the adult front teeth that erupt somewhat irregularly. This space is called “Leeway Space”.

C. Schematic View of Leeway Space

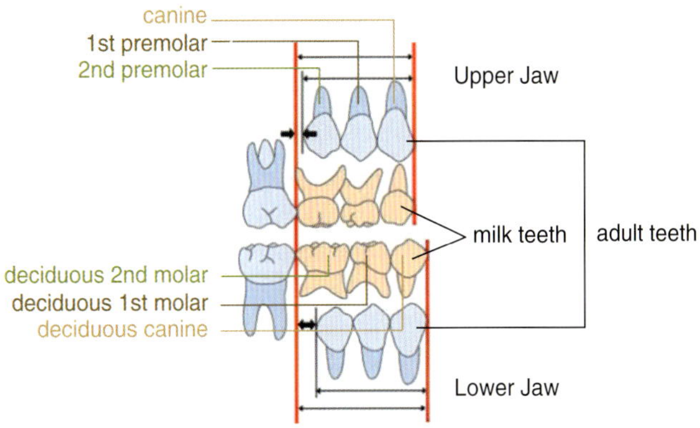

Yellow colored teeth are deciduous canine, 1st molar, and 2nd molars(milk teeth) which are appeared in the oral cavity and the blue colored teeth are canine, 1st premolar, and 2nd premolar which are adult permanent teeth located underneath the deciduous teeth within the alveolar bone.

D. Improper Eruption Order Can Result in a Snag Canine

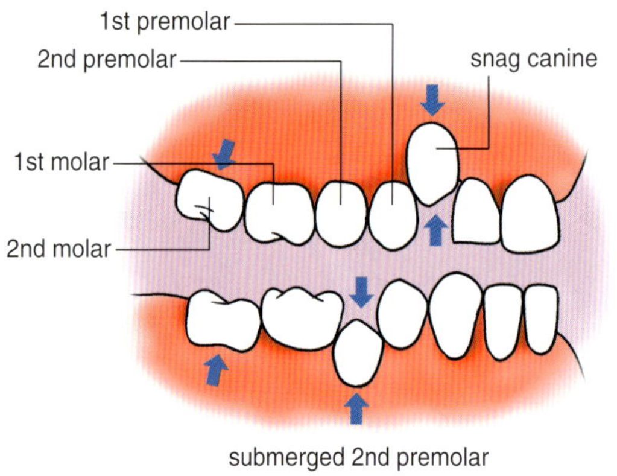

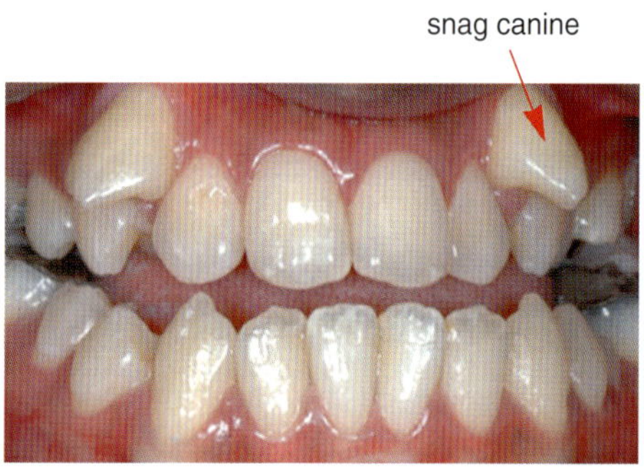

Adult canine is the strongest and most stable of all the teeth with a single long root and a pointed tip. It resembles the tooth of Carnivora whose action is to tear the flesh of the prey. Hence it is called the name canine.

Because they are positioned in the corner of the mouth, they have an important role of maintaining the shape of the lips which is very important factor for facial esthetics. Upper canine erupts after the complete eruption of the incisors(front teeth) and premolars (small-sized back teeth). Thus, the lack of space can often lead to snag canine of upper jaw. Whereas, lack of eruption space in the lower jaw causes the 2nd premolar to be submerged.

E. Discomfort Induced by Snag Canine

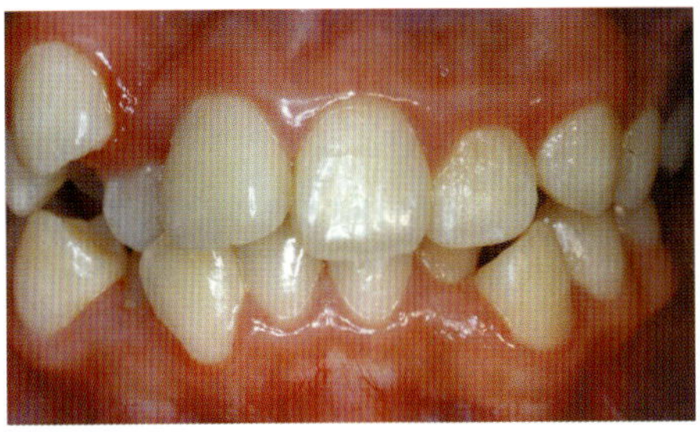
before treatment of snag canine

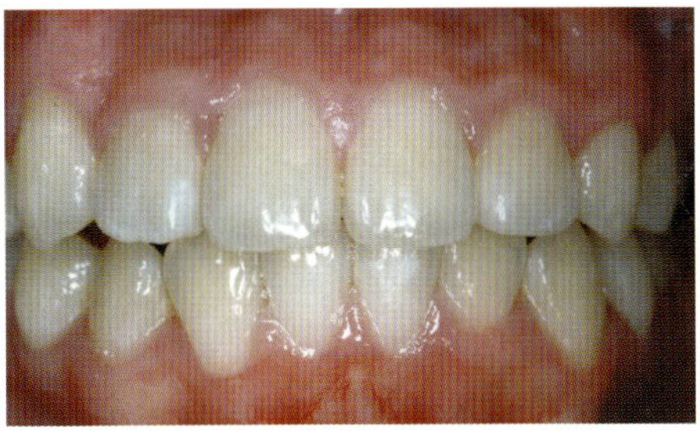
after only one year treatment

The patient who has snagged canine complains that it can easily tear the inner skin of the lip while vigorous activities such as wrestling, climbing, basketball, and icy hockey. Having snag canine is similar to having a sharp stone in the mouth. And upper lips frequently get stuck while laughing and speaking.

F. Even the Ancient Scholars Detested the Bad Alignment of Teeth

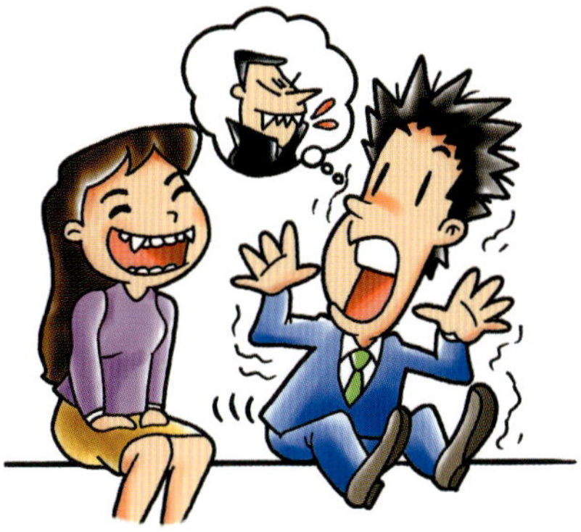

The negative view toward badly aligned teeth goes all the way back in history to ancient times. Literary works of ancient scholars such as Hippocrates, Aristotle, Celsus, and Pliny all commented on an alignment of teeth.

It is well known that Hippocrates was among the first to comment about dental problems as follows;

Among those individuals with long shaped heads, some have thick necks, strong parts and bones. Others have strongly arched palates, their teeth are irregularly arrayed, crowding one another, and they are bothered by headache and discharge from the ear(otorrhea).

Celsus, Aurelius Cornelium(1st century AD), a celebrated Roman medical encyclopedist noted that teeth could be moved by finger pressure.

Adamandios, the Greek philosopher of 5th century AD, noted that "those persons whose lips are pushed out because of cuspid displacement are ill-tempered, abusive shouters and defamers.

Similar negative views on snag teeth still are widespread among Americans and Europeans whose culture inherited from the ancient Greek civilizations.

G. Could the Prime of Youth Cover the Handicap of Snag Canine?

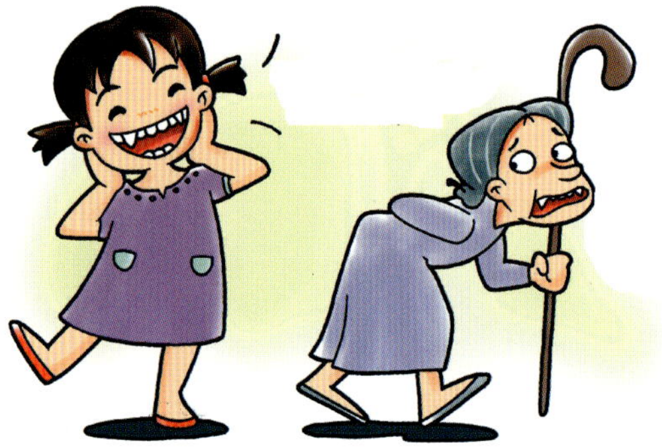

There are some opinions that snaggletooth among teenagers and people in their early 20s are considered to be cute. But this could only apply to people at a young age. People in their 30s, 40s, or 50s with snaggletooth can be perceived by others to have an unpleasant, often terrifying look. This is because snaggletooth definitely do not look good with wrinkled face. This suggests an extra reason why treatment of snaggletooth for aging people is quite necessary.

15. Treatment of Snag Canine

A. Moving the Molar Teeth Backwards

B. Lateral Expansion of the Upper Jaw (Palatal Expansion)

C. Examples of Orthodontic Treatment by Using Rapid Palatal Expander

D. Moving the Front Teeth Forward

E. Undersizing the Front Teeth (Interdental Disking)

F. Extraction of Premolars

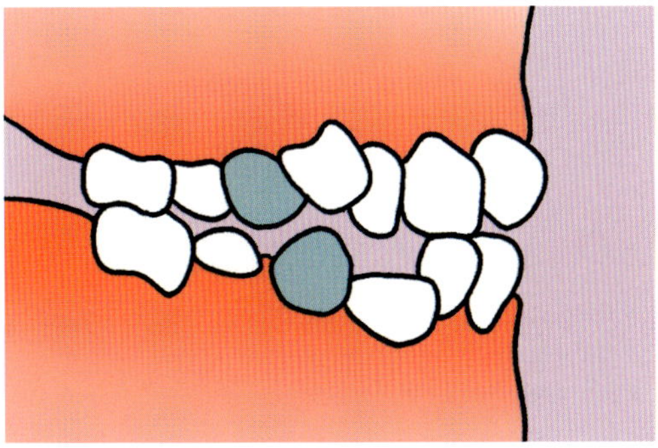

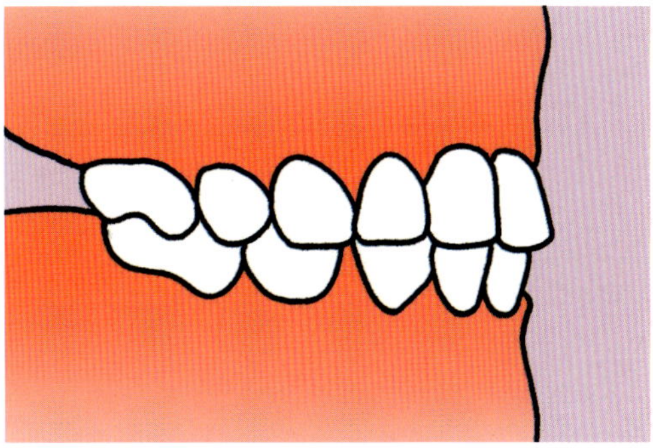

A. Moving the Molar Teeth Backwards

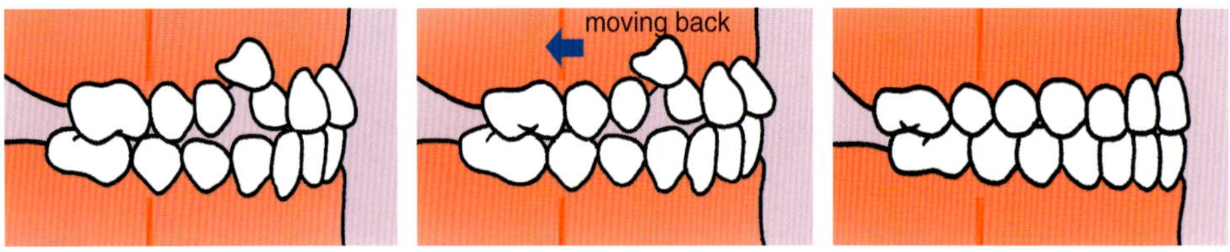

before treatment under treatment after treatment

The first option is attaining the space by moving the back teeth (molars) to the further back. However, current orthodontic skills only allow 2~3mm movement of the last molar teeth, which provides less than half the space for proper alignment of the snaggled canine.

B. Lateral Expansion of the Upper Jaw (Palatal Expansion)

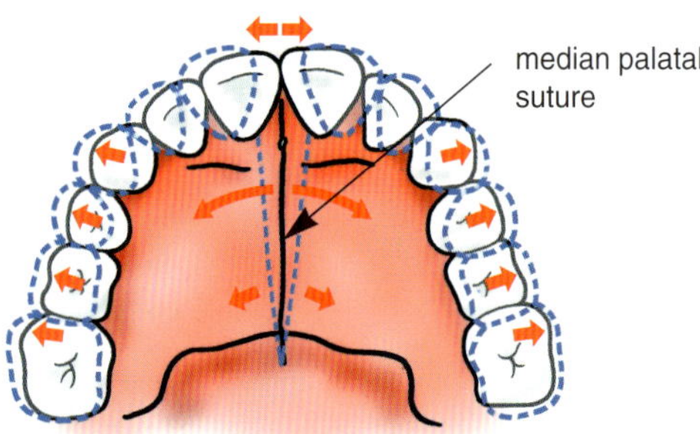

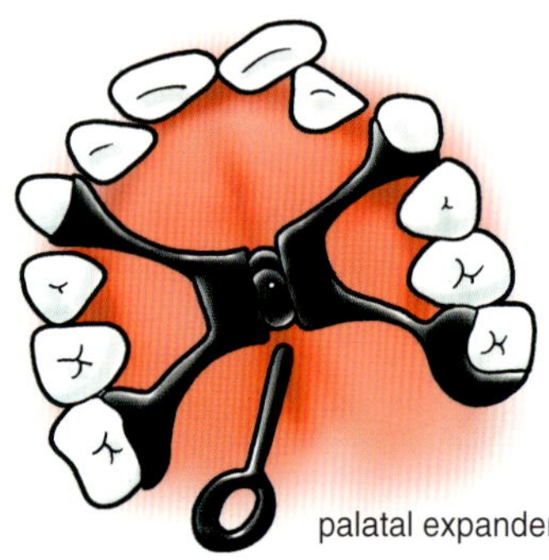

palatal expander with screw key

The second approach involves expanding the upper jaw laterally using appliance named "Rapid Palatal Expander". The upper jaw is made up as if the two joint parts are sealed together which is called "median palatine suture". Thus, if strong tearing force is applied through the use of orthodontic appliance, Palatal Expander, the jointed two parts will separate apart.

However, because the sealing of both sides becomes very rigid as one ages, they cannot be separated simply by the use of orthodontic appliances after adolescence. Therefore, a special dental surgery such as corticotomy is required for adult patients.

Thus, this method is only viable for young children who have bad relationships between upper and lower teeth due to a very narrow width of upper jaw.

C. Examples of Orthodontic Treatment by Using Rapid Palatal Expander

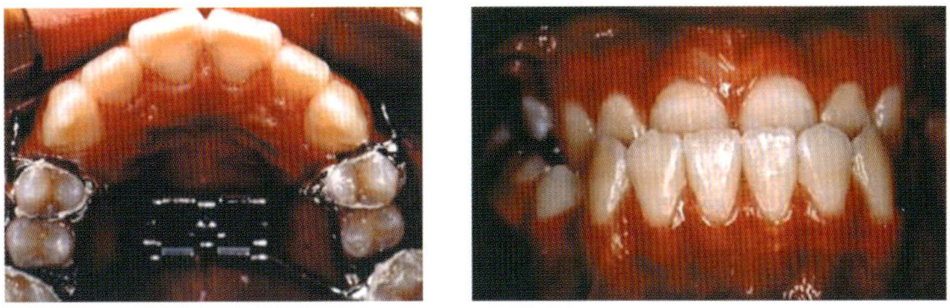

before treatment

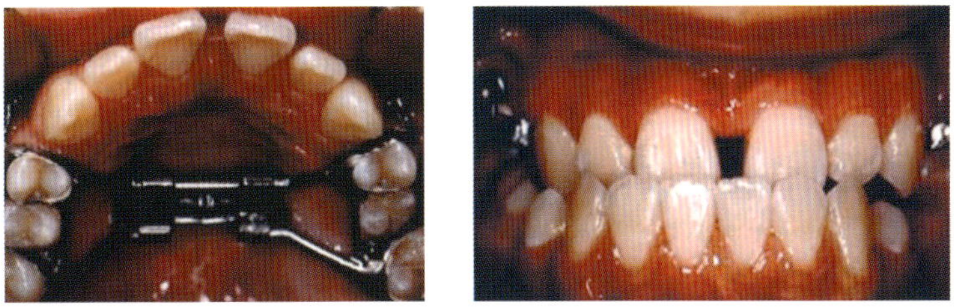

under treatment

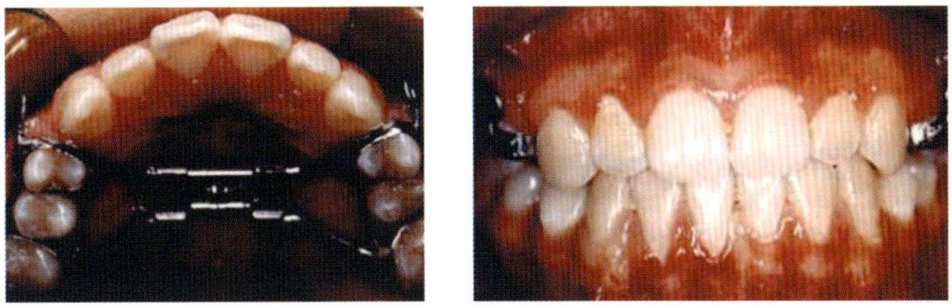

after treatment

D. Moving the Front Teeth Forward

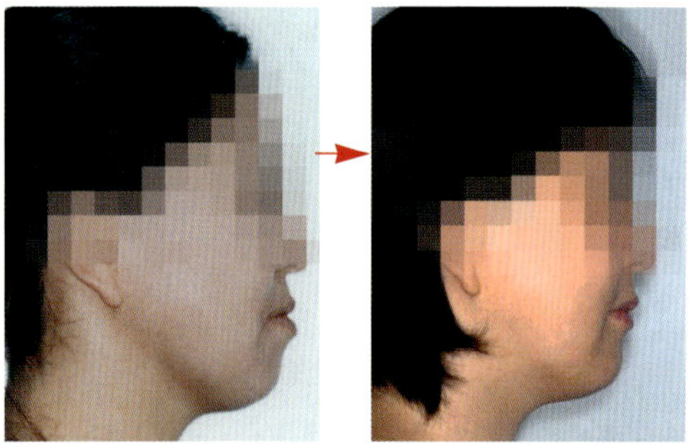

Treatment without extraction results in damaging effect such as protruded lip(left photo). So, four premolars are removed for improvement in facial esthetics(right).

It is possible to move the front teeth forward for properly aligned dentition. Treatment without removing any adult teeth improves only the alignment of teeth, but the front teeth are tilted forwards making the mouth form into the shape of a monkey's.

Obviously, this can seriously damage one's looks. In this case, the premolars(small-sized back teeth) should be removed.

E. Undersizing the Front Teeth (Interdental Disking)

Space for good alignment of snag canine teeth also can be created by undersizing the teeth width called "interdental disking". Undersizing the crown width by getting rid of tooth material between the teeth can be another approach. However, the maximum space available from this method is no more than 4mm.

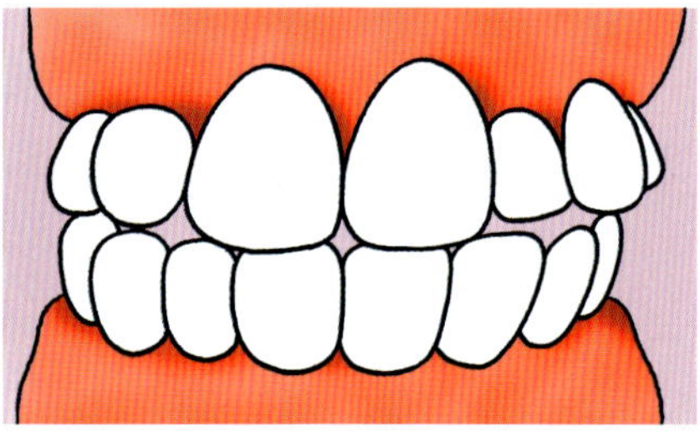

Irregularly aligned front teeth

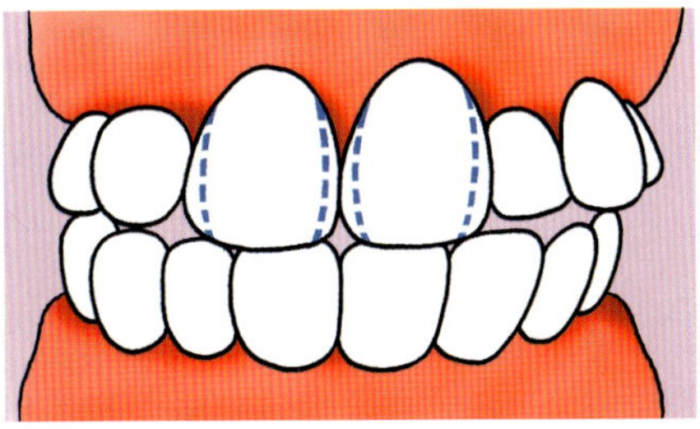

Extra space is gained by grinding in-between the teeth with sand paper

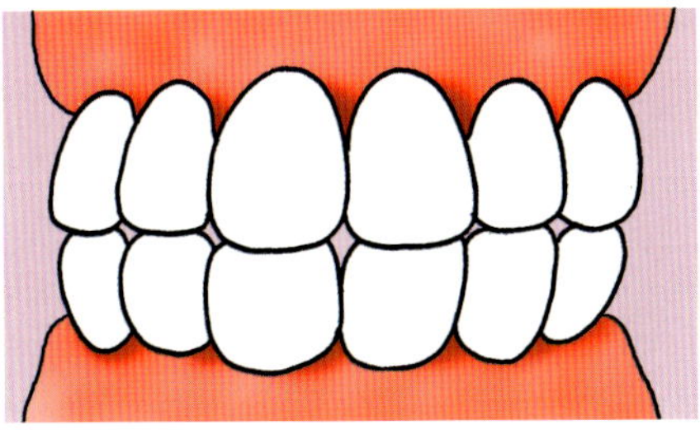

Alignment of the teeth after treatment.

F. Extraction of Premolars

Space can be obtained by extracting premolars. Extraction almost always is required to obtain enough space if space deficiency is 10mm or more.

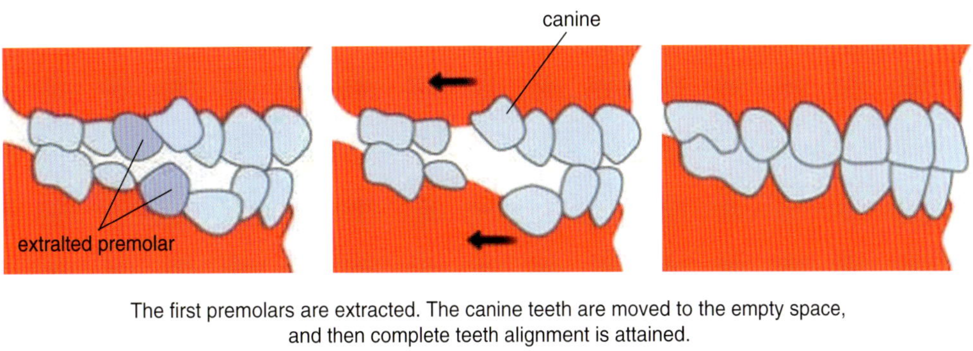

The first premolars are extracted. The canine teeth are moved to the empty space, and then complete teeth alignment is attained.

16. Maxillary Protrusion

A. Protruding Front Teeth with Revealed Gum

B. Main Causes of Maxillary Protrusion

C. The Front Teeth of the Lower Jaw Bites the Palate.

D. Showing the Gum while Smiling

E. Difficulties in Swallowing

F. Difficulties in Closing Lips

G. Protruding Teeth Causes Gum Diseases

H. Difficulties in Pronunciation

J. Higher Risk of Fracturing Upper Front Teeth

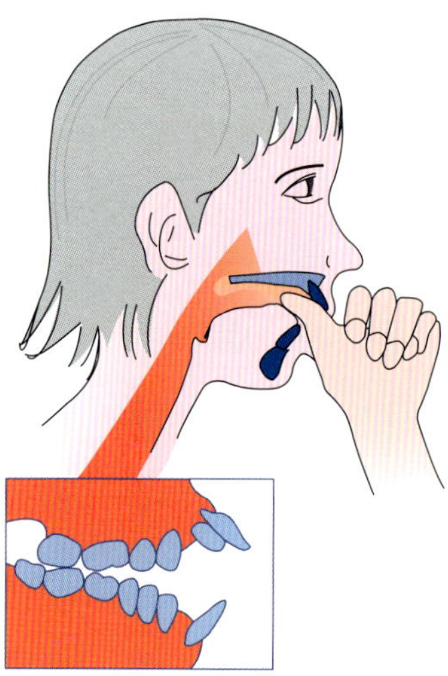

A. Protruding Front Teeth with Revealed Gum

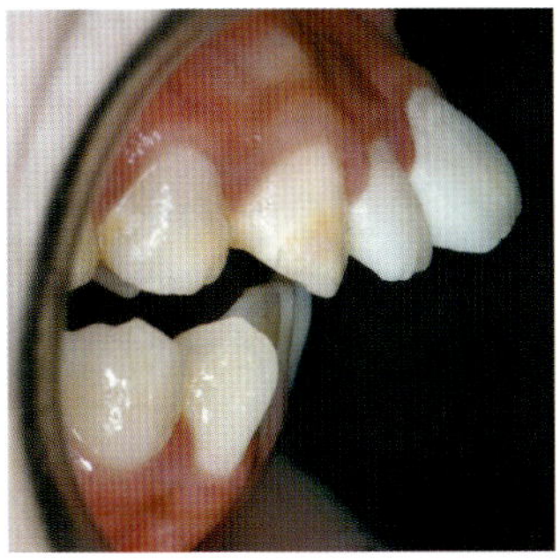

Protruded upper jaw including teeth are referred to as maxillary protrusion.

There are various types of maxillary protrusion;

1. Badly tilted upper front teeth.
2. Upper teeth that are positioned in the front part of the upper jaw.
3. Both upper and lower teeth are positioned in the front part of the both jaw.
4. Extremely long upper jaw resulting from small amount of growth in the lower jaw.

B. Main Causes of Maxillary Protrusion

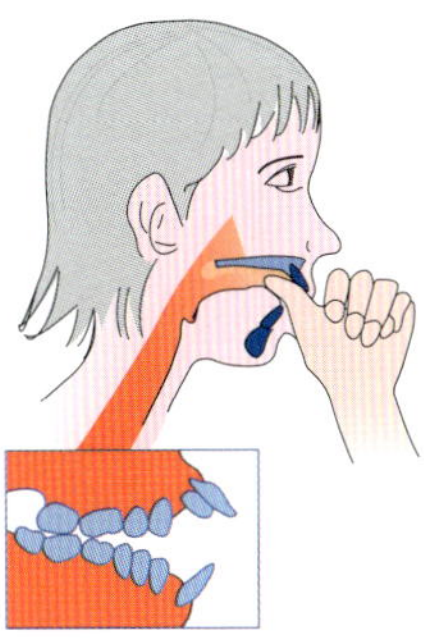

Maxillary protrusion among children can be caused by finger sucking. These children often have a gap between the upper and lower front teeth.

Also, maxillary protrusion can be found among those with a habit of sucking lower lips or those who always breath through the mouth resulting from a stuffy nose.

Recent research revealed that a fetus tends to suck his/her fingers when feeling bored.

C. The Front Teeth of the Lower Jaw Bites the Palate

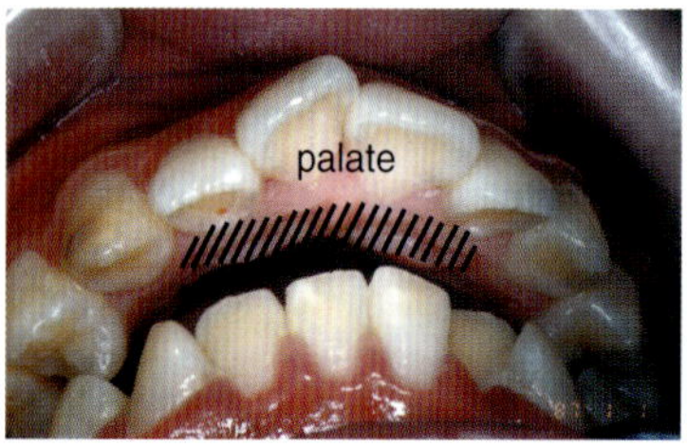

before treatment

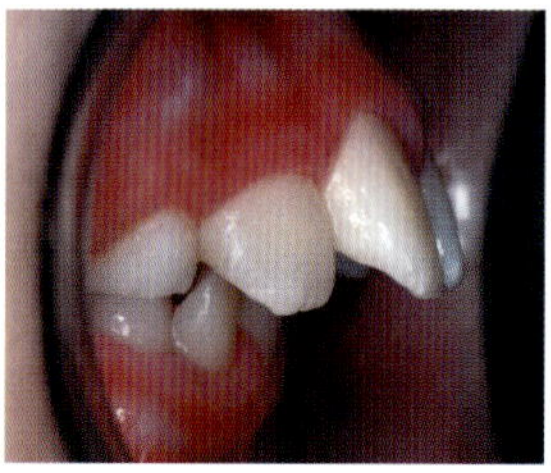

lateral view

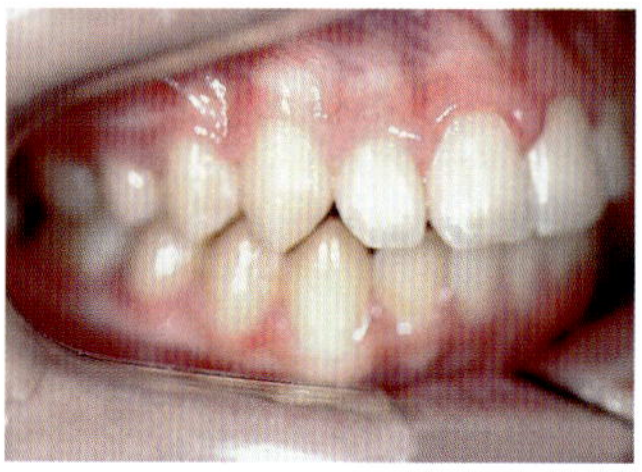

after treatment

Distinguishing maxillary protrusion is relatively easy. If the front teeth of the lower jaw are completely covered by those of upper jaw, or if the front teeth of lower jaw touches the gum of the inner side of the front teeth(palate) of the upper jaw, it can be said that the patient is suffering from serious maxillary protrusion. Because the lower teeth constantly apply pressure to the root of the upper front teeth, it could damage the front teeth of the upper jaw.

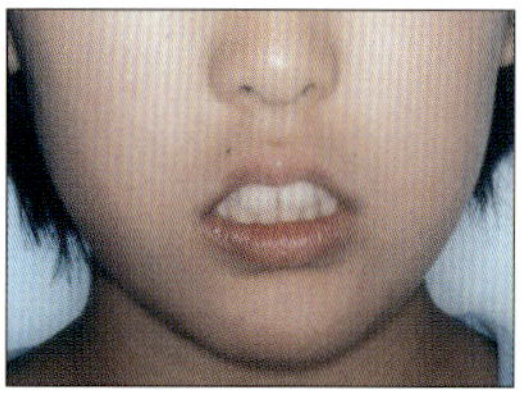

lip in resting position

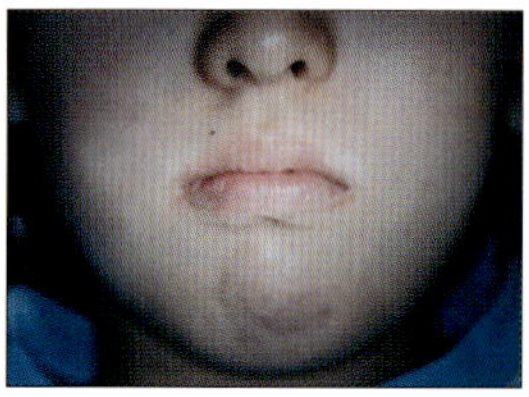

strained lip

Abnormal lip shape in case of maxillary protrusion

Usually, patients of maxillary protrusion tend to stick out the lower jaw forward intentionally when asked to close the mouth. Therefore, for a precise examination, orthodontists should ask the patient to swallow saliva first and then to have the mouth closed.

D. Showing the Gum while Smiling

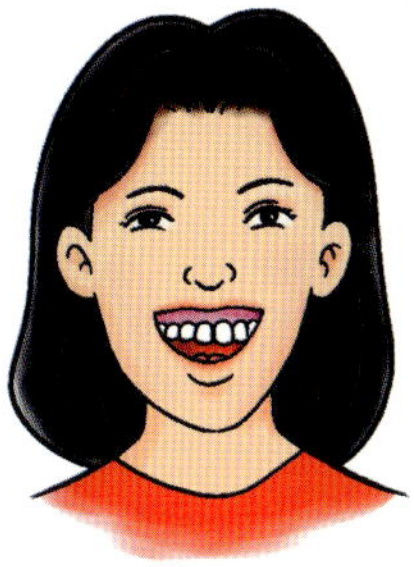

gummy smile before treatment

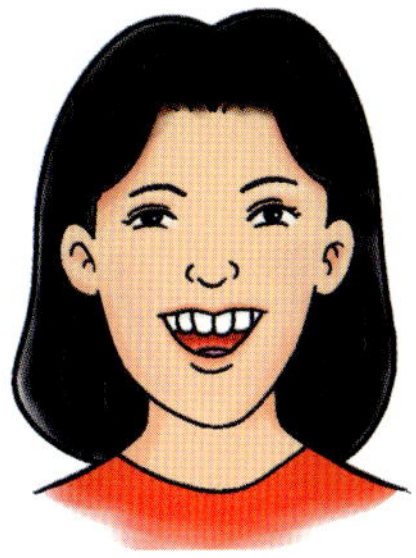

after treatment

Maxillary protrusion can be noticed just by looking closely at someone's mouth. People with protruded upper jaw tend to open their mouth slightly when they are in resting state.

Some parents misunderstand this symptom and think that maybe this is caused by their children's unusually short distance between the nose and the upper lip.

If the children often open their mouth and then their upper front teeth is revealing while watching TV, or gums are shown excessively when they smile, it can be concluded that the children suffers from serious maxillary protrusion.

E. Difficulties in Swallowing

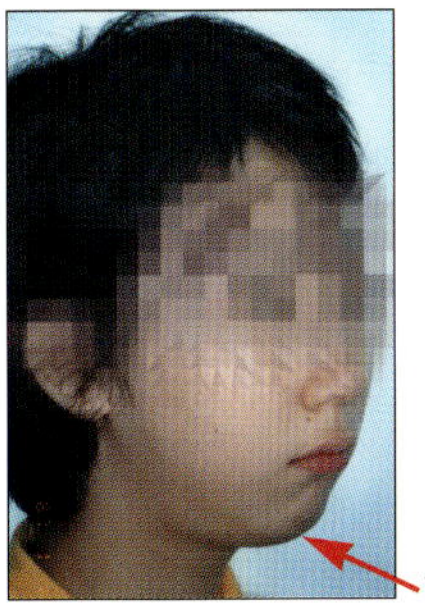

walnut-shell like wrinkles

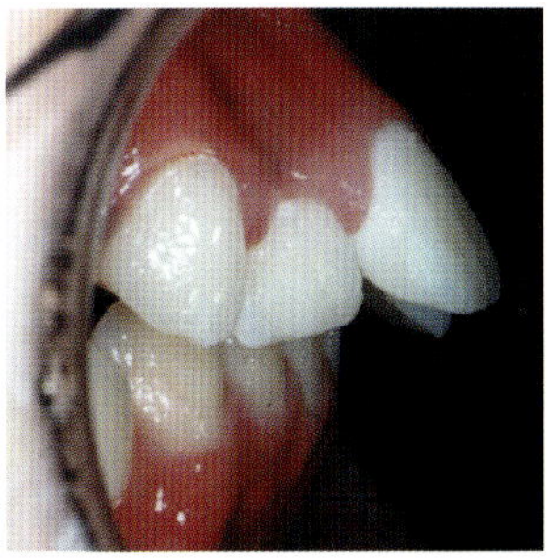

Maxillary protrusion can be noticed by the way a patient swallows his/her saliva. Patients whose front teeth are severely protruded will have to stretch out their tongue in order to make a vacuum in mouth whenever they swallow something. When this patient swallows saliva or food, muscles surrounding the lips excessively strains, thus dimples, that looks similar to walnut shells, are formed on the lower chin.

F. Difficulties in Closing the Lips

With protruded upper jaw, it is hard to close the lips properly. Therefore, lips can become very dry. In such cases, one must wet the lips with the tongue to speak continuously.

They usually put extra effort in closing the lips in order to hide their protruded upper front teeth. However, while they are taking a rest or sleeping, the muscles surrounding the lips are released and the front teeth are spontaneously shown.

It is quite easy to imagine a person with this problem dozing off in the bus or subway with his/her mouth open and drooling.

G. Protruded Teeth Causes Gum Diseases

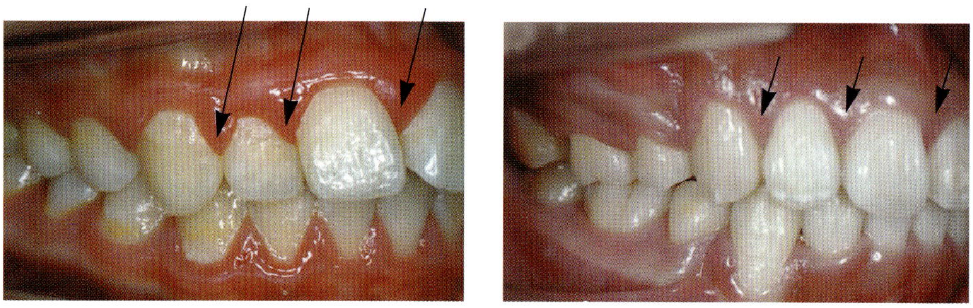

Arrows indicate diseased gum before treatment. Right photo shows normal healthy gum after treatment.

Saliva functions as a natural sterilizer in the mouth. An opened mouth dries the saliva coated on the gums. As a result, gums can be easily exposed to various bacterial attack, resulting in gum diseases.

When viewed closely, healthy gums should show small protrusions called stippling and the color should be coral pink.

On the other hand, infected gums are often glittering and show reddish. In such cases, people with this problem often bleed in the mouth while brushing their teeth or biting into hard food stuffs such as apple or hamburger.

H. Difficulties in Pronunciation

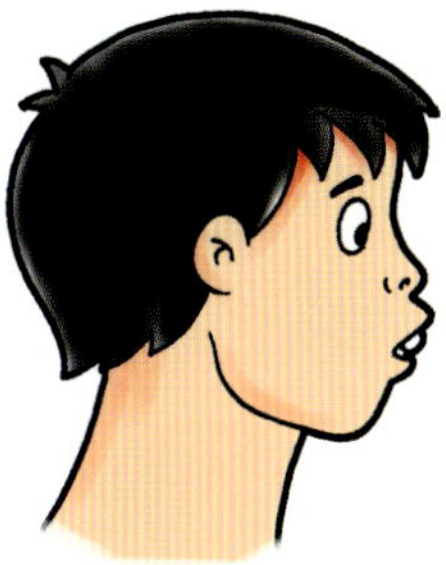

In some cases, pronunciations with the letters "s" or "b", require the use of both teeth and lips. Severely protruded upper front teeth make it difficult to close the mouth, and this can lead to serious burdens when pronouncing certain words.

And because it is hard to close his mouth properly, he would often find himself spitting to others while talking. Also, these people find it extremely hard to swallow saliva naturally, and this can lead to the bad habit of talking too fast.

I. Higher Risk of Fracturing Upper Front Teeth

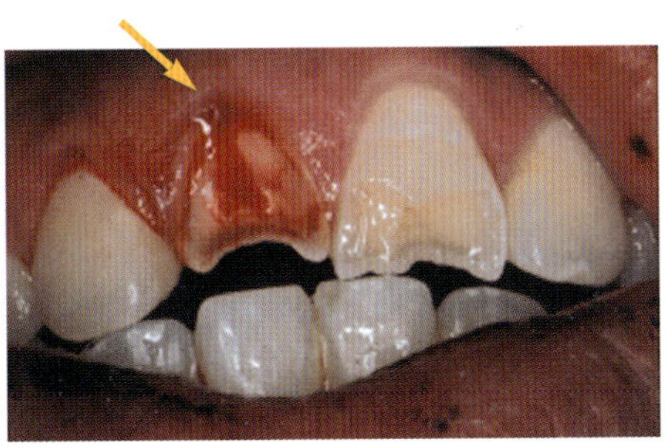

fractured upper front teeth

In addition, a person with protruded upper front teeth has a higher risk of fracturing during a car accident or a sports-related accident.

17. Treatment of Maxillary Protrusion

A. Headgear

B. How Does the Head Gear Work?

C. Extractions Combined with Headgear

D. Treatment by Functional Appliance such as Twin Block

E. Examples of Gummy Smile Treatment by Combination Therapy

F. Examples of Gummy Smile Treatment by Botox and Filler

G. Cheerful Outlook on Life after Treating Protruded Upper Jaw

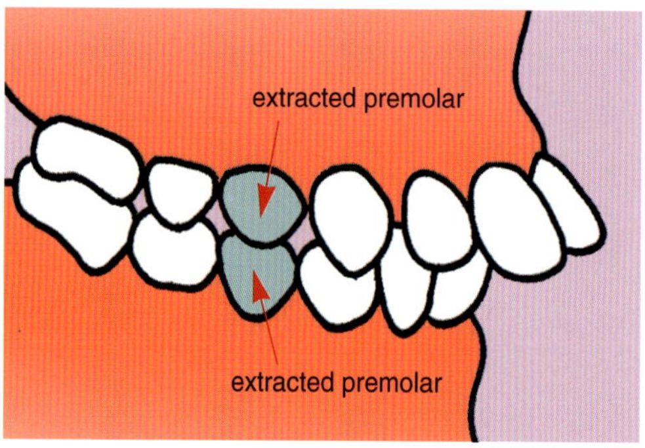

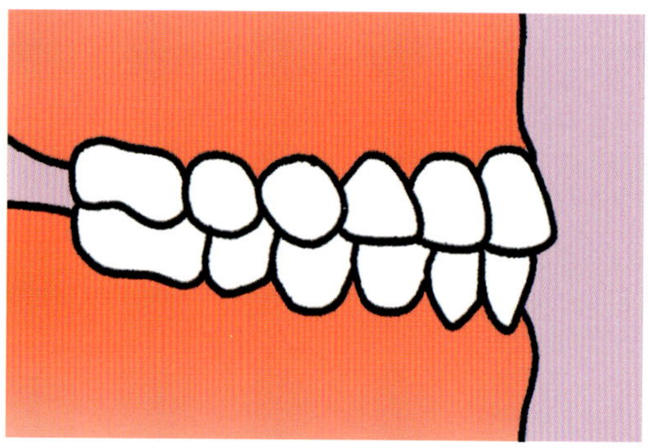

A. Headgear

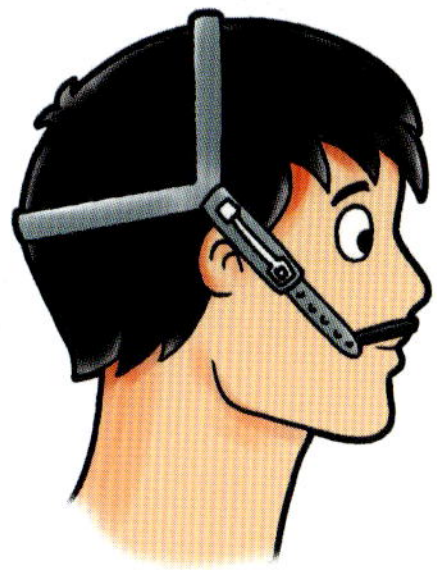

A person with a headgear on

Neglecting the treatment of maxillary protrusion during adolescence can lead to the relatively rapid growth of the upper jaw compared to the lower jaw. As a result, the already protruded upper jaw can become even more severe after growth. In such cases, using a headgear will prevent the abnormal overgrowth of the upper jaw.

B. How the Head Gear Works.

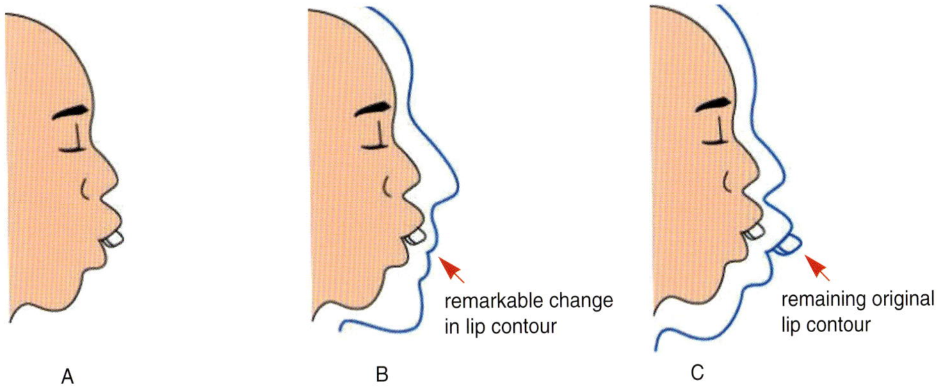

A. Before treatment.
B. With the aid of a headgear, the contour of the upper jaw changed properly.
C. Neglecting wearing the headgear will make the situation worse.

C. Extractions Combined with Headgear

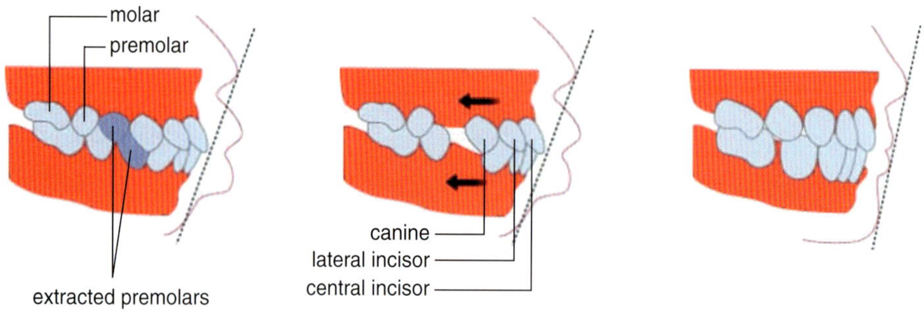

A B C

A. Before treatment

B. To treat the protruded upper and lower jaw, four premoalrs were removed, then the six front teeth (4 incisors and 2canines, totally 6 teeth) are pushed back, and the back teeth (premolars and molars) are kept in the original position by way of anchorage using headgear or mini pin placement.

C. Results of a successful treatment with the help of a headgear or mini pin.
Unfaithful use of a headgear can leave gaps between the upper and lower front teeth. Recently mini pin is widely used for effective treatment. Mini pin can make it almost unnecessary to wear headgear.

D. Treatment by Functional Appliance such as Twin Block

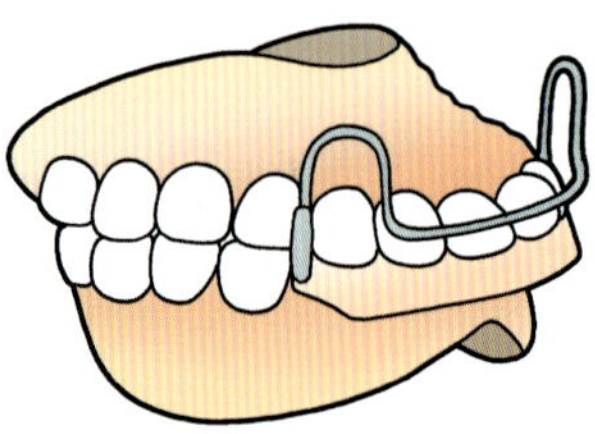
Functional Appliance

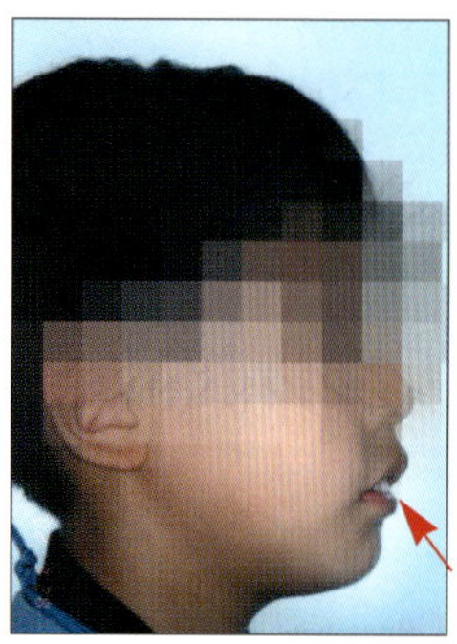
before treatment

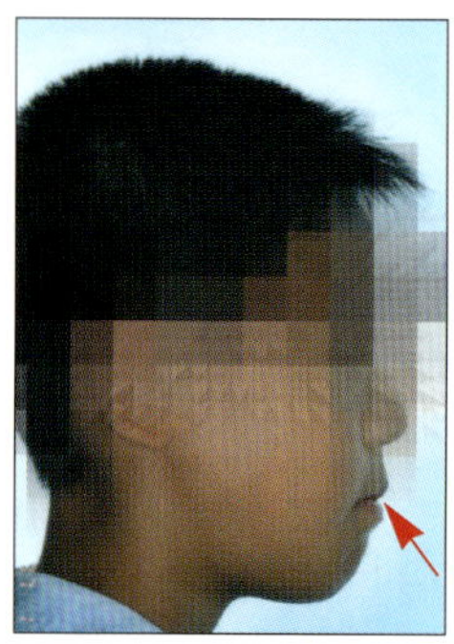
after treatment

Because of protruded upper teeth, he is unable to close his mouth. The horizontal distance between upper and lower front teeth is over 10mm. Eight months after the treatment with a Twin Block is shown on the right end photo. His facial appearance is changed, and is able to close his mouth easily.

E. Examples of Gummy Smile Treatment by Combination Therapy

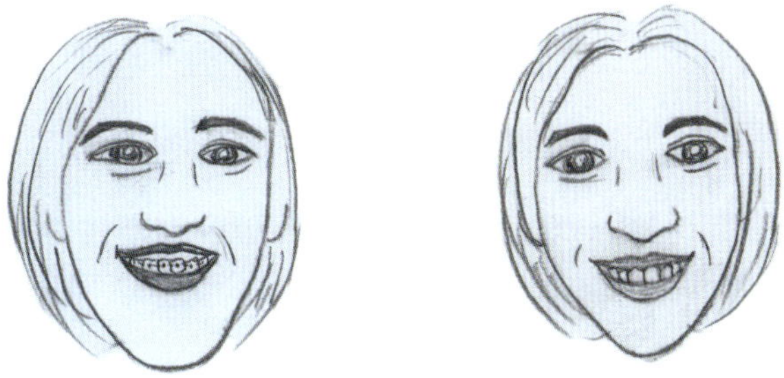

before treatment after combination therapy

If one's upper teeth and gums are severely protruded, the upper lip cannot cover the entire set of teeth properly. Thus, when they smile, their gums are inevitably revealed. Such a smile is sometimes referred to as a "gummy smile", and it is considered to be very unattractive among people. Combination therapy with orthodontic treatment and surgery enables her smile to look natural.

F. Treatment of Gummy Smile Treatment by Botox and Filler

Botulinum toxin is often produced by growing in improperly handled or prepared meat products and described as sausage poison. The word "Botulinum" is originated from a latin word "botulus", meaning sausage.

Botulinum toxin is the most poisonous neurotoxin ever discovered. In December 1989, Botox manufactured by Allergan, Inc, was approved by FDA for the treatment of strabismus(crossed eyes), blepharospasm (uncontrollable blinking of eyes), and hemifacial spasm in patients over 12 years old. Also used for treating spasm of the lower esophageal sphincter and inhibiting the over sweating. Botox is now used for various cosmetic and medical procedures.

Canadian Doctors firstly used Botox for treating forehead frown lines. After formal trials, FDA announced regulatory approval of Botox to temporarily improve the appearance of moderate-to-severe frown lines between the eyebrows. Subsequently cosmetic use of Botox becomes widespread.

Recently botox is widely used in dentistry for treating slight gummy smile. Side effects were deemed to be rare, mild and treatable.

The results of cosmetic effects vary but can last up to eight month. Thus, patients are required to re-inject two or three times a year.

G. Cheerful Outlook on Life after Treating Protruded Upper Jaw

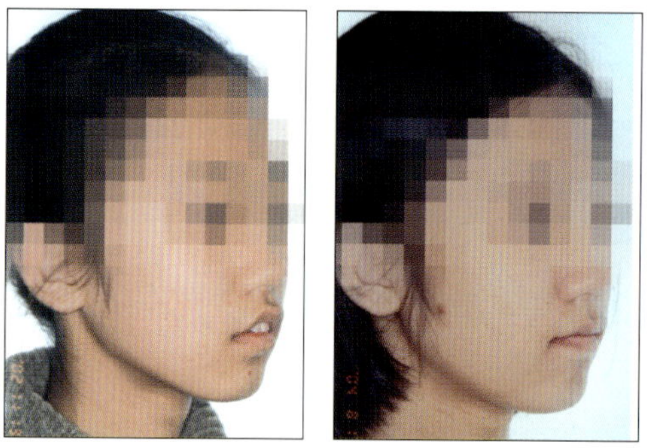

before treatment after treatment

This patient must give an extra effort to close the lips. Tension around the lips are generated in order to close the lips. In the state of relaxation, lips are opened and the front teeth are revealed(left). After treatment, the external lip contour is corrected normally and it enables this person to close her mouth naturally.

After the treatment, some patients found themselves feeling confident about their looks. She now puts on make-up and pays close attention to how she dresses and is so happy that she is confident in meeting other people. All in all, her perspective toward life has changed.

18. Anterior Openbite

A. Definition

B. Causes

C. Openbite Treatment by Tongue Crib

D. Gap Between the Upper and Lower Front Teeth Causes the Person to Frown during Swallowing

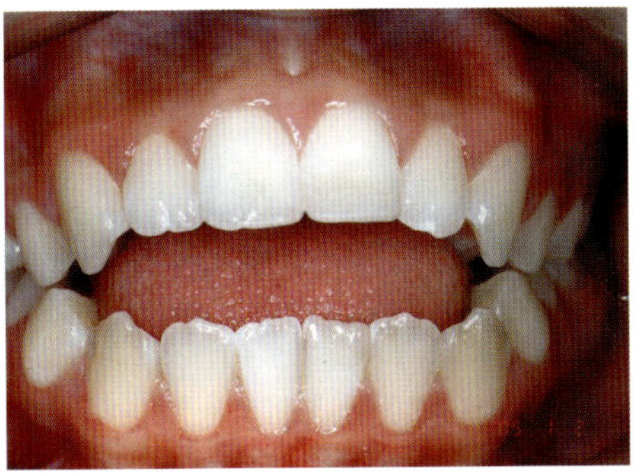

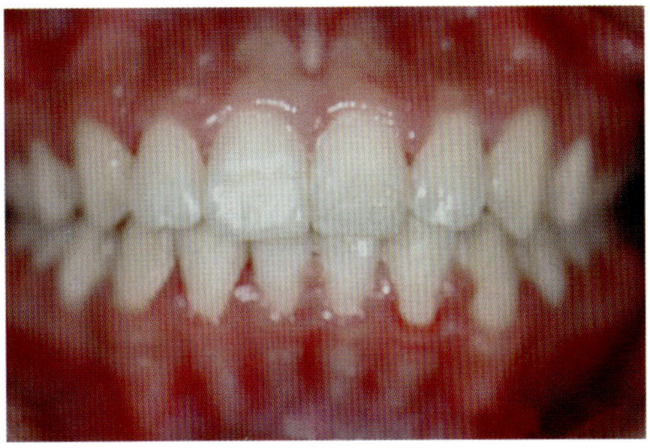

A. Definition

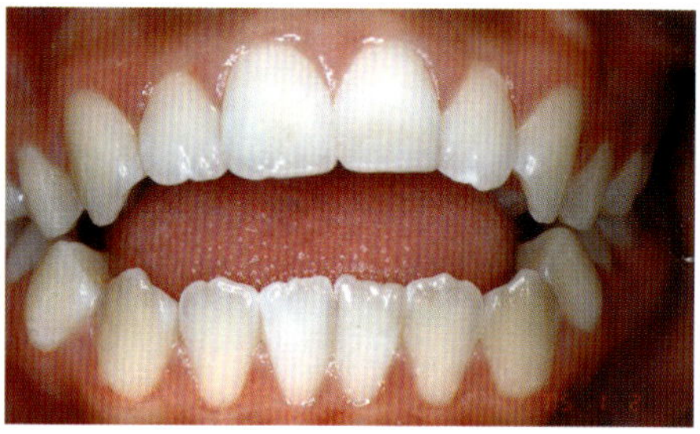

before treatment

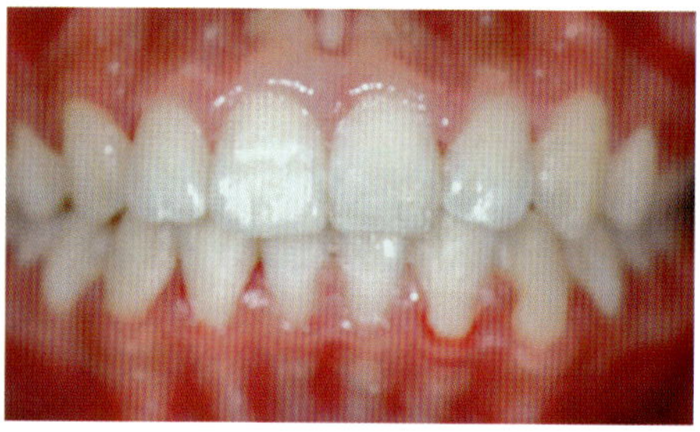

after treatment

An anterior openbite is defined as the condition where the front teeth of upper and lower jaws are not in contact with each other when the both jaws are closed.

B. Causes

One of the main causes of anterior openbite lies with an improper location and function of the tongue, sucking fingers, swollen tonsils, acute pharyngitis and cerebral palsy which is caused by the malfunction of the brain.

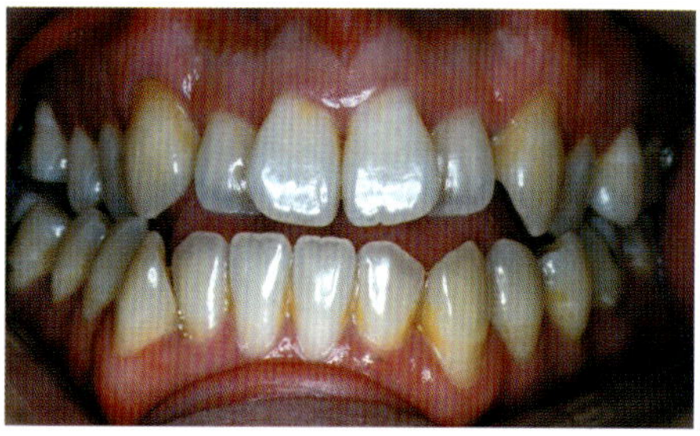

Before treatment

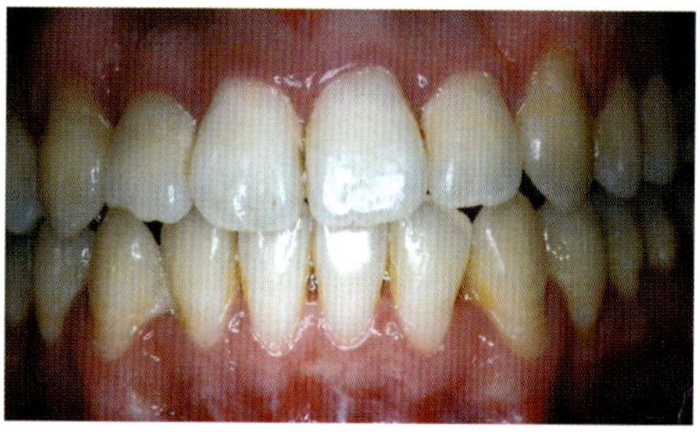

Combination therapy
with orthodontics and surgery was done

C. Openbite Treatment by Tongue Crib

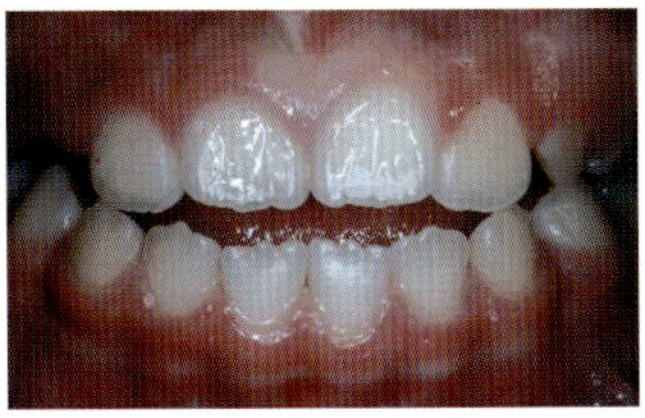
before treatment

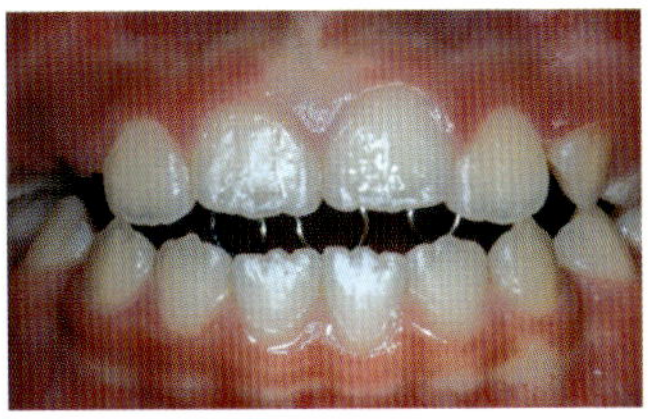
wearing tongue crib

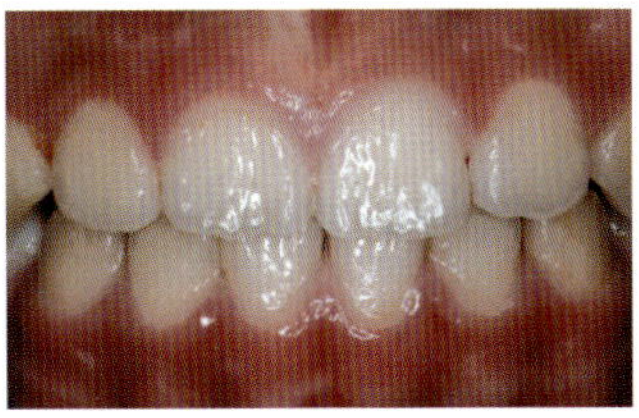
after treatment

Thumb sucking habit results in anterior openbite. Tongue crib is used for solving this problem.

D. Gap Between the Front Teeth Causes the Person to Frown during Swallowing

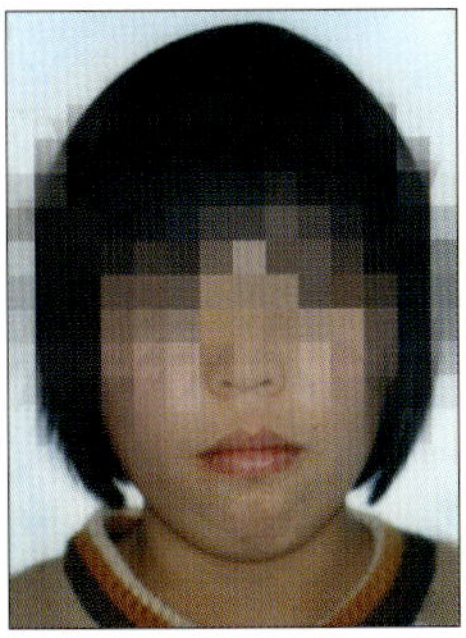
before treatment

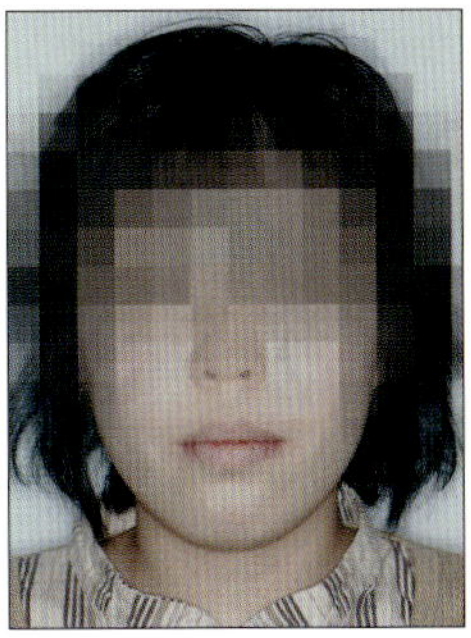
after treatment

In case of anterior openbite, swallowing something contracts the muscles surrounding the mouth in order to stabilize the lower jaw, and this causes the person to frown whenever he swallows because of unstable condition of the lower jaw.

A slight gap between the upper and lower front teeth would not significantly affect the shape of the face. However, severe anterior openbite will cause excessive tension to the lips since the person applies extra pressure while closing his mouth. Also, openbite weakens the bite force of the front teeth due to the gap between the upper and lower front teeth.

In addition, people with anterior openbite commonly reveal their tongue during conversation and this often leads to the mispronunciation of the words.

19. Diastema (Space between the Upper Front Teeth)

A. Expels Good Fortune

B. Ugly Duckling Stage

C. Spontaneous Disappearance of Diastema after Canine Eruption

D. Supernumerary Teeth

E. Abnormal Labial Frenum

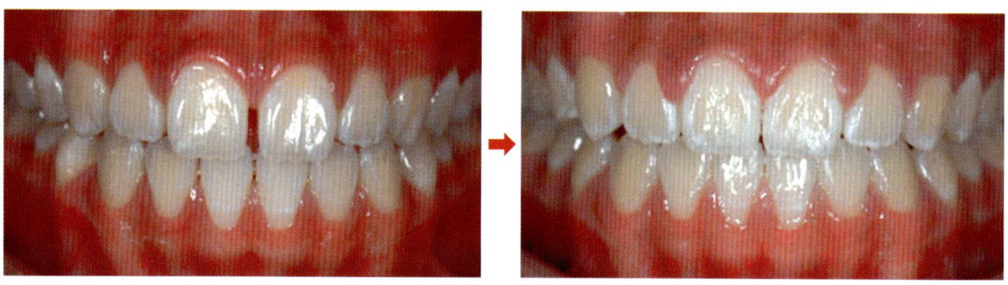

A. Expels Good Fortune

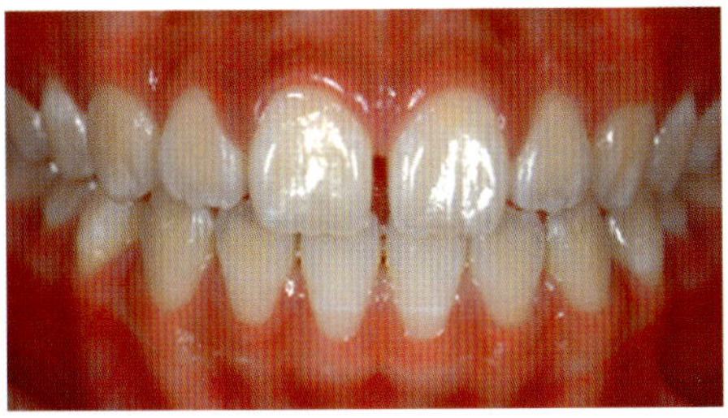

before treatment

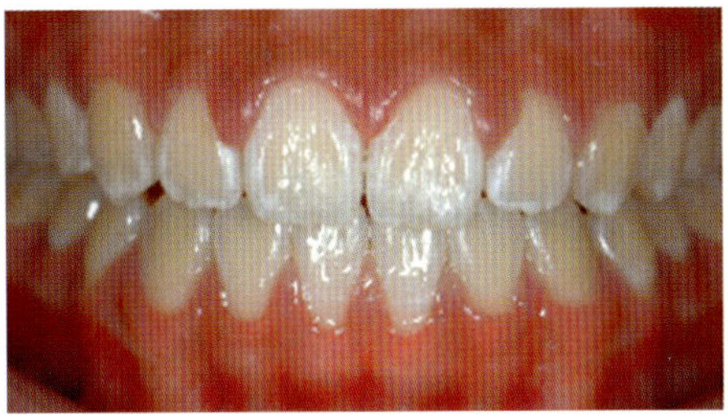

just after treatment

In this case, if the treatment will be done by artificial teeth (prosthesis), it looks rather unnatural and with the lapse of a certain amount of time, the treatment needs to be done over again.

Diastema is the condition where a space exists right in the middle of the front teeth on the upper jaw. Our ancestors abhorred this appearance since they believed that a space between the front teeth of upper jaw would enable good fortune to leak out, and that is the main cause of receiving treatment.

People with severe diastema are easily noticed by others. There are no particular problems concerning pronunciation and chewing, but these people can appear as if they lack seriousness in daily lives.

B. Ugly Duckling Stage

In most cases, adult front teeth of the upper jaw are neatly aligned and have point to point contact. However, in spite of normal growth process in one's childhood, the front teeth of the upper jaw shows a space.

Such examples can be seen when canines inside the alveolar bone exert pressure to the root of the front teeth(central and lateral incisors). Usually, diastema disappears when the canine begins to erupt.

Such phenomena is a part of the natural developmental process of childhood. However, in Western countries, this period is commonly referred to as the "ugly duckling stage" of

Andersen's fairy tale, since this phenomena takes place when children least listen to their parents. In other words, this is an essential stage that children must go through to become a pleasant looking adult.

C. Spontaneous Disappearance of Diastema after Canine Eruption

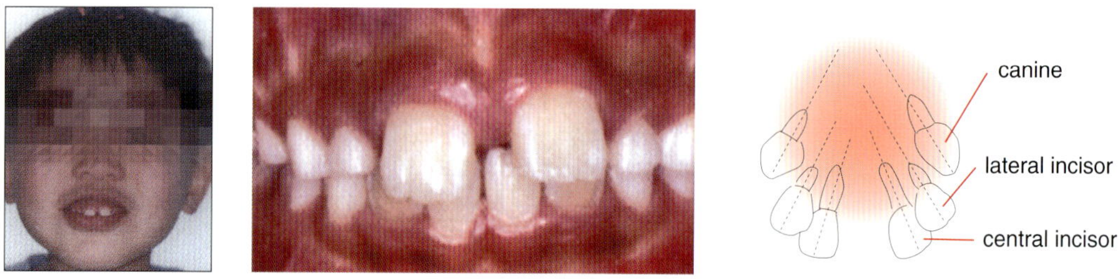

Canine, that is growing in the alveolar bone is pressing the root of two front teeth(central and lateral incisors), enabling a space to appear between the upper front teeth.

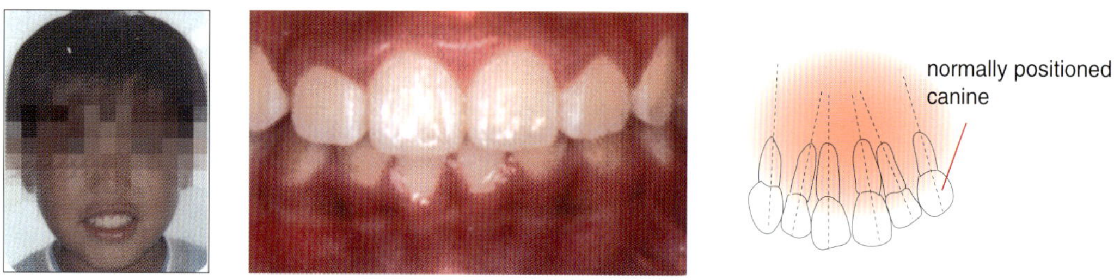

As canine erupts, the space begins to reduce. Completely erupted canine at the age of about 10 leads to properly aligned teeth. No treatment was given at all.

D. Supernumerary Teeth

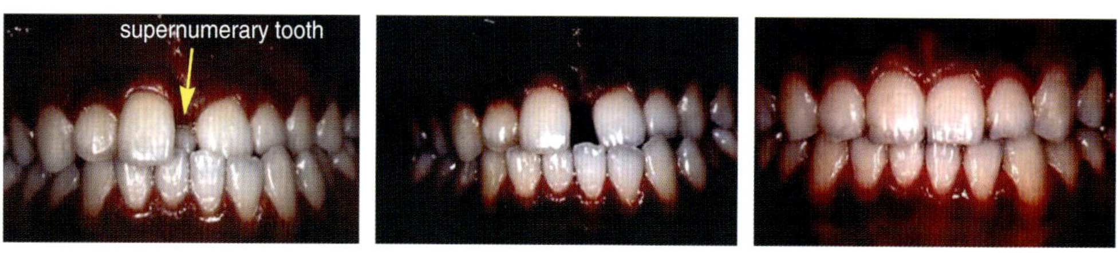

before treatment | just after removal of supernumerary tooth | after treatment

In some cases, a space exists between two central incisors of the upper jaw, due to an impacted extra tooth lying between the central incisors. This state can easily be observed by an X-Ray exam and the lying extra tooth must be removed in its early stages. Orthodontic treatment is necessarily required for disappearing this space.

E. Abnormal Labial Frenum

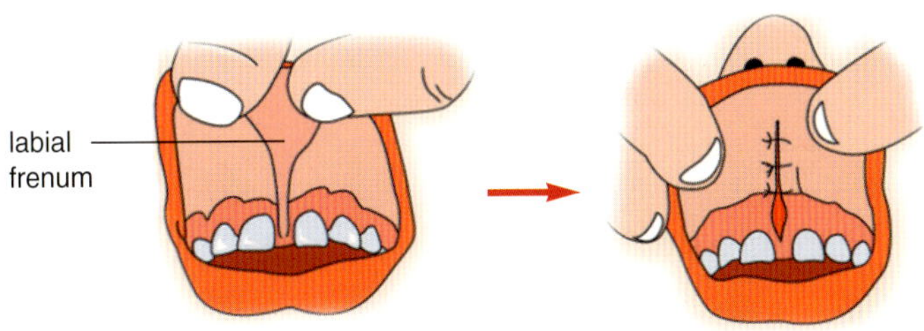

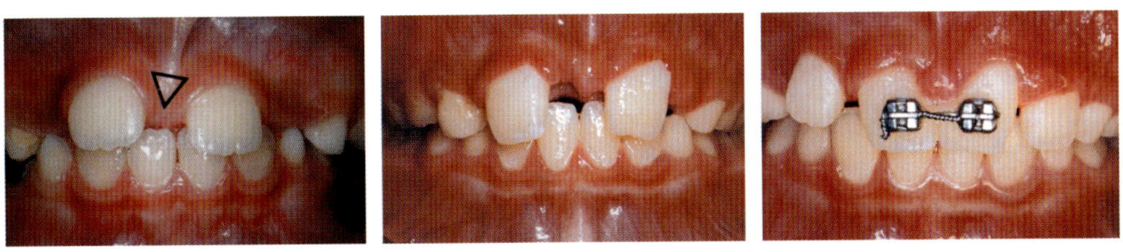

Over-extended tough labial frenum is surgically cut, sutured(frenectomy), and orthodontic treatment was done.

If the labial frenum of upper jaw extends to the inner side of the front teeth, it must be removed at once in order to close the space between the teeth before orthodontic treatment begins.

20. Sparsely Aligned Teeth

A. Space between the Teeth

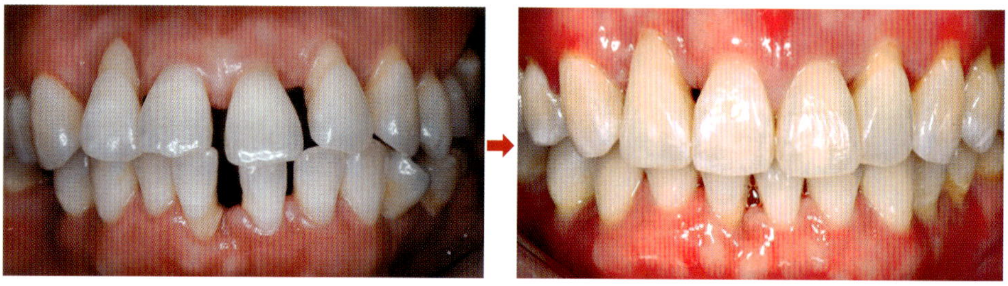

A. Space between the Teeth

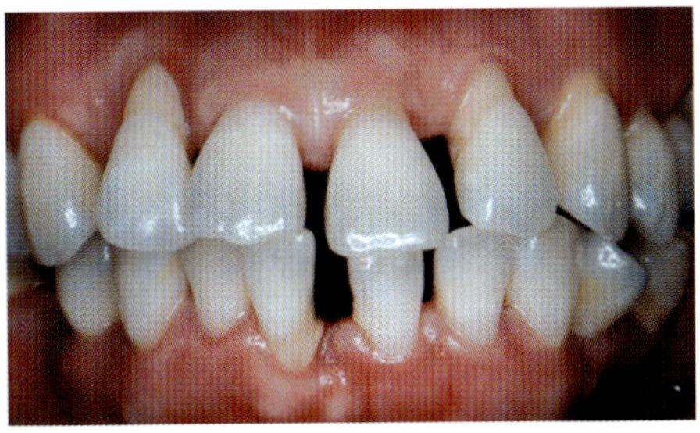

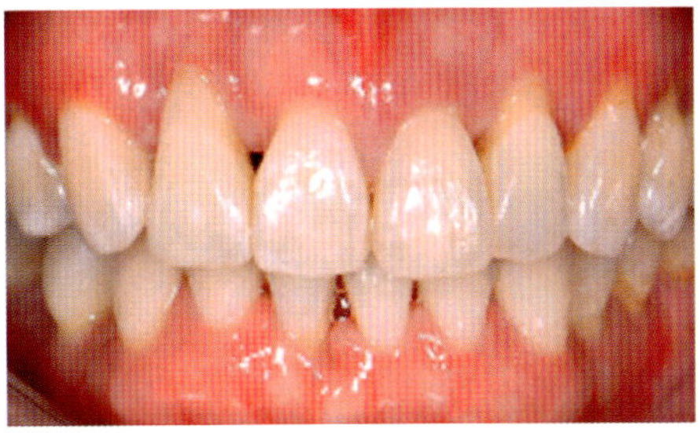

Space between the front teeth can be noticed easily. The space has been completely closed after treatment. The patient was satisfied with the treatment. Prosthetic(crown) treatment can shorten the treatment period. However, over-sized teeth look rather unnatural. Moreover, the treatment must be repeated every 7~8 years.

Not only do the sparsely aligned teeth look ugly, but they also can cause a speech impediment. In some Asian countries, it has long been believed that such a sparsely aligned teeth bring misfortune. Also, improperly aligned teeth cause a person to spittle while talking.

An increasing number of people are now seeking treatments for the front teeth since a good impression is known to be important when meeting others and making friends. Sparsely aligned front teeth should be treated since they are easily noticeable by others, especially during conversation and smiling.

21. Special Circumstances

A. Posterior Openbite

B. Locked Upper One Tooth

C. Facial Asymmetry

A. Posterior Openbite

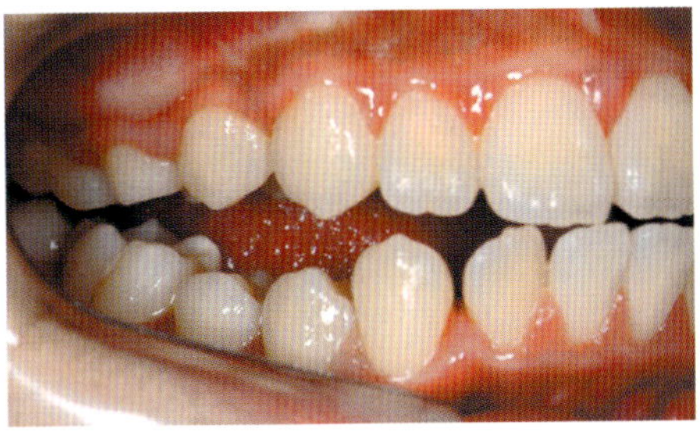

A: before treatment

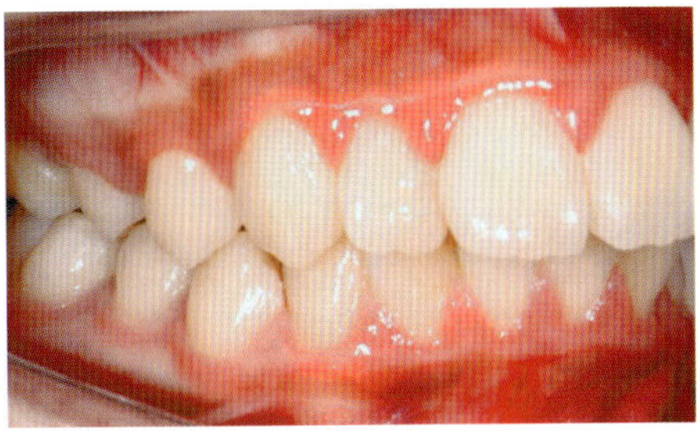

B: after treatment

Posterior openbite which is very rare could be caused by lack of eruption of back teeth(molars).

B. Locked Upper One Front Tooth

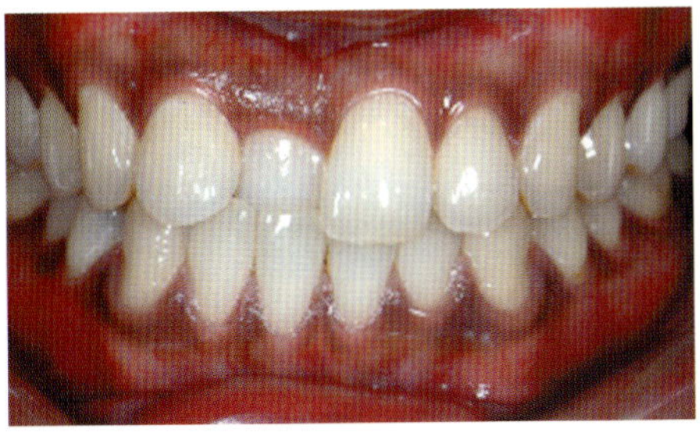

before treatment

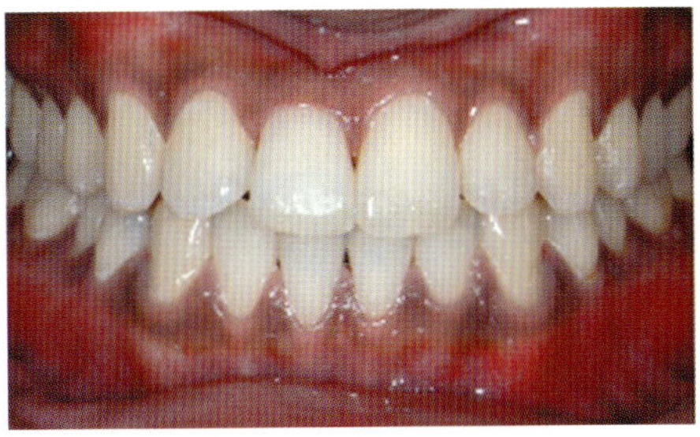

after six month treatment

C. Facial asymmetry

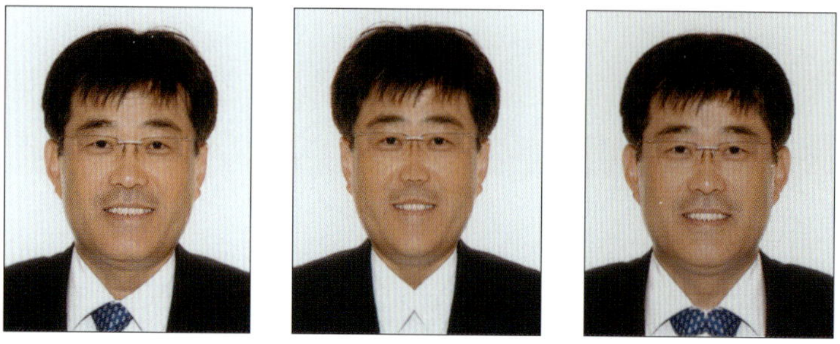

A　　　B　　　C

A: Original photograph
B: Composite of the two left sides of the picture
C: Composites of the two right sides of the picture

A slight degree of bilateral facial asymmetry exists even in normally looking individuals. This can be revealed most readily by comparing the real full face photograph with composites consisting of two rights or two lefts sides.

22. Mandibular Prognathism (Long and Tilted Lower Jaw)

A. Habsburg Royal Family

B. Long and Tilted Lower Jaw Is Inherited from the Parents.

C. Long and Tilted Lower Jaw Brings Good Fortune?

D. Having Difficulties in Eating and Speaking

E. Symptoms Begin to Show at an Early Age

F. Difference between Adult and Infant in the Shape of Temporomandibular(Jaw) Joint

G. Artificial Deformation of Bone Structure

H. Head Deformation of Incan People

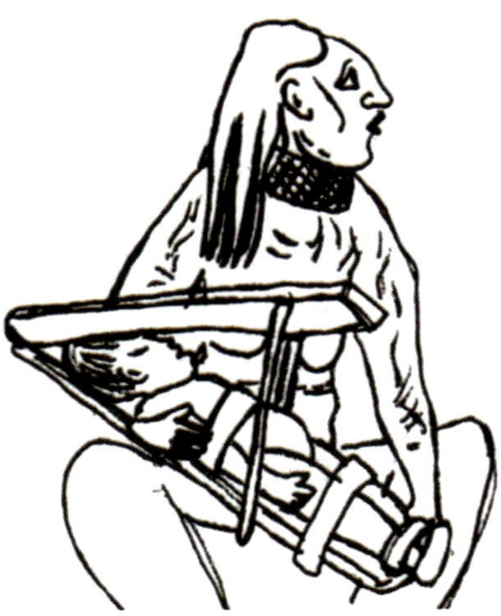

A. Habsburg Royal Family

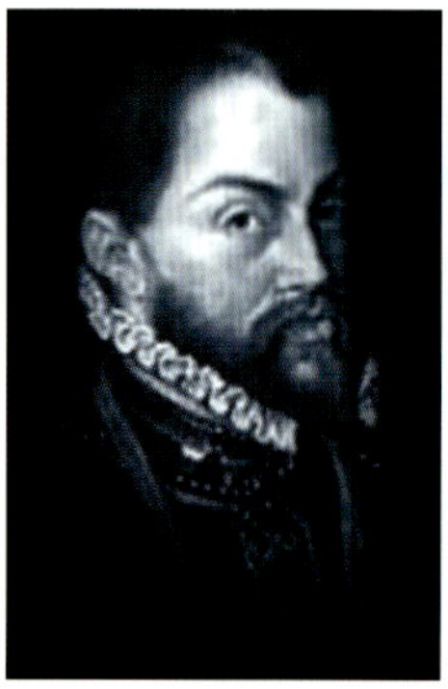

Portrait of Rudolf II.
He could not keep his mouth shut because of long and tilted lower jaw. Fries occasionally entered his mouth, so he had to grow a beard.

This is the portrait of Royal Families of Habsburg, who set the medieval European dominion under their control. In order to conquer Spain, Austria, German, and other European Empires, consanguineous marriages were engaged. As a result, most offsprings had long and tilted lower jaw, and this became the symbol of the Habsburg Royal Families. Most of the offsprings had to suffer from long and tilted lower jaw.

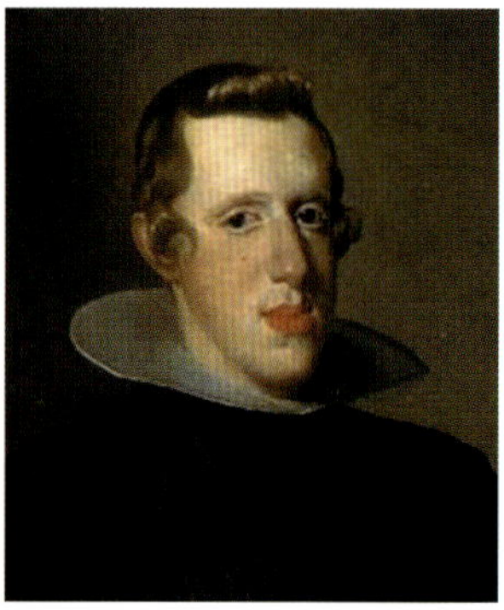

Portrait of King Philip IV.
He always salivated, and could not chew properly. He died of general weakness in the end.

Philip the IV seemed to have no problem while young; however, it became worse as he aged. Severely long and tilted lower jaw resulted in drooping spit constantly. Also he could not speak properly and had problems in chewing and swallowing.

B. Long and Tilted Lower Jaw Is Inherited from the Parents

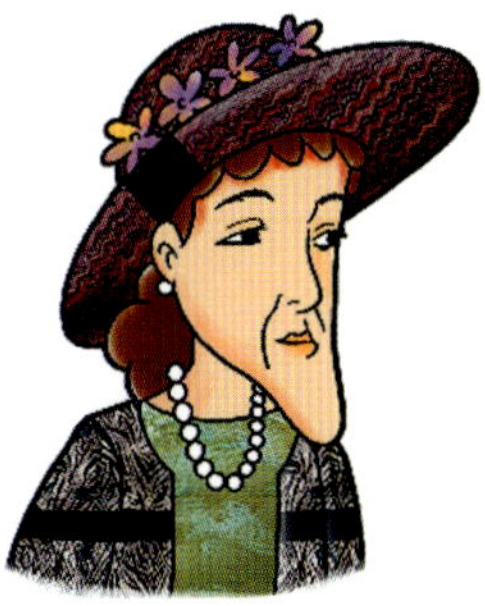

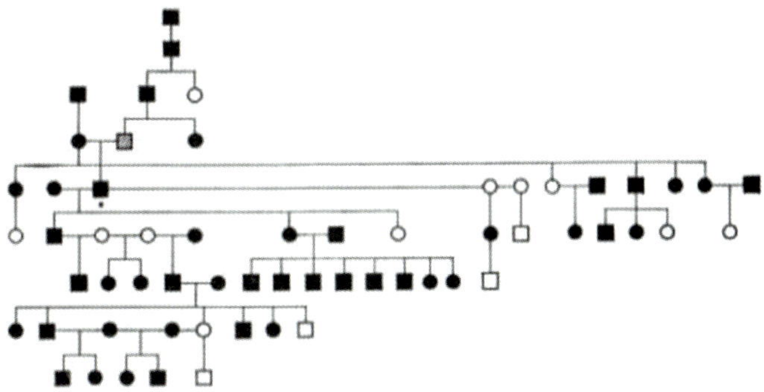

Pedigree of Hapsburg Royal Family. Blank is normal, and black is long and tilted lower jaw. Square is male, round is female.

If a family member has a long and tilted lower jaw, the chances of having a same type of lower jaw later on increases. Therefore, it is important to consult with an orthodontist regarding this matter.

In view of human life, the tendencies of abnormal direction of jaw growth can not be changed reversely on the way, thus there is no chance for protruded upper jaw to become a long and tilted lower jaw tendencies on the contrary later on.

C. Long and Tilted Lower Jaw Brings Good Fortune?

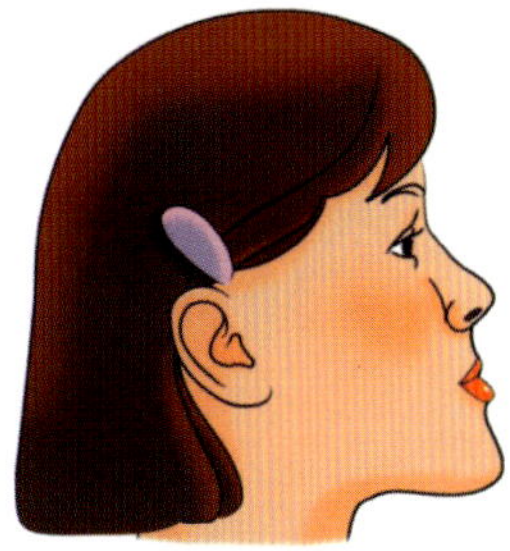

The typical long and tilted lower jaw

Because the lower jaw is long and tilted, the feature of the face may give a strong and powerful impressions, and it looks like a big rice scoop, long and big jaws were considered to bring good fortune to a family for a long time in Korea.

However, in modern times nobody can honestly feel happy about having this type of jaw, especially to the women. Actually, the belief about bringing good fortune was merely a fictitious story generated during times when cosmetic surgery for long jaws was not possible.

D. Having Difficulties in Eating and Speaking

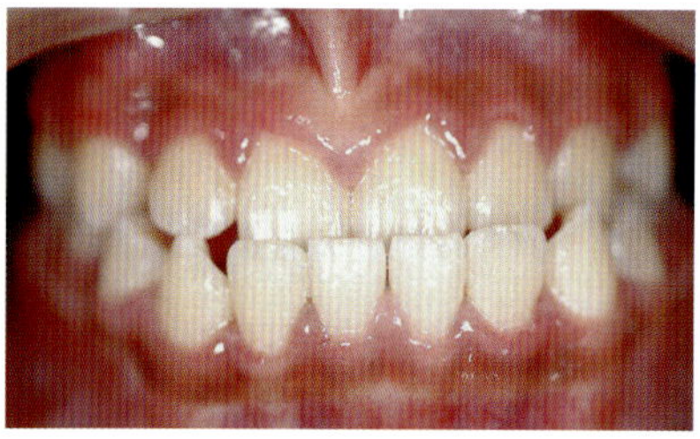

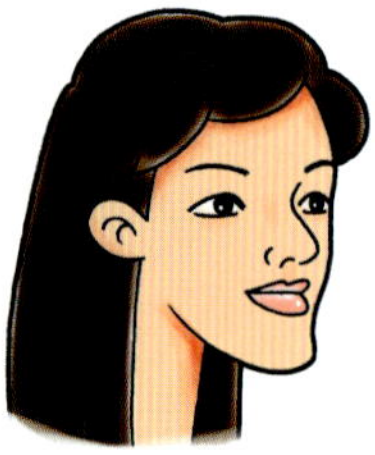

For the normal chewing function, the lower teeth are covered by upper teeth. A person with a tooth alignment like this photo cannot chew properly. It takes extra effort in eating, and food often falls out of the mouth. Even swallowing saliva is difficult for these people with over-extended lower jaws. Bulldogs and cats have similar jaw structures and it can often be seen that these pets spill out food around the dish.

Also exact pronunciation of words become difficult, especially words with the letters "f" and "v". For such people, the most burdening factor could be the ugly appearance that results from a long and tilted lower jaw.

E. Symptoms Begin to Show at an Early Age

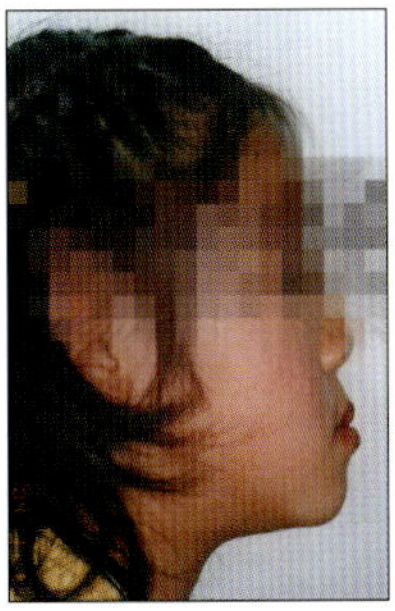
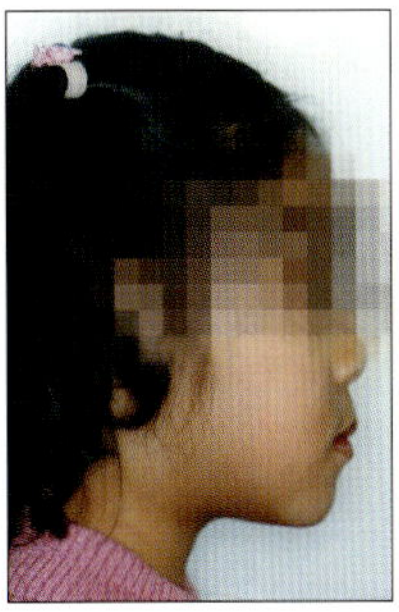

profile change

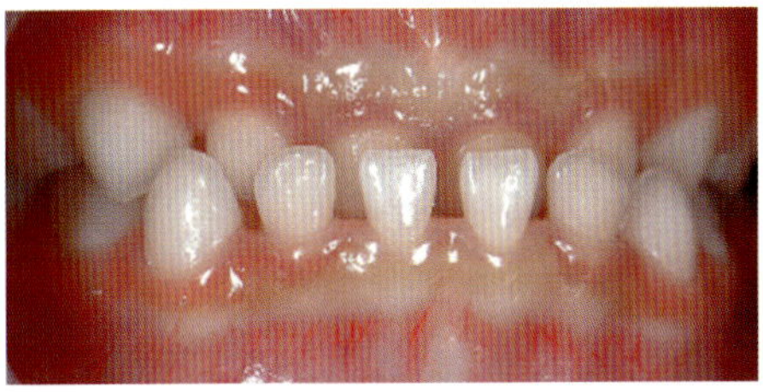

before treatment

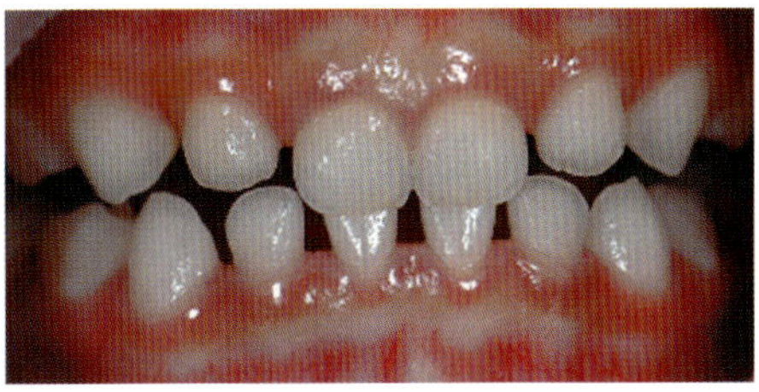

after treatment

Infants between 6~12 months old only have front teeth and in some cases their lower front teeth cover the upper front teeth. Normally the upper set of teeth should cover the lower ones. So their worried mothers visit dentists for some answers.

F. Difference between Adult and Infant in the Shape of Temporomandibular(Jaw) Joint

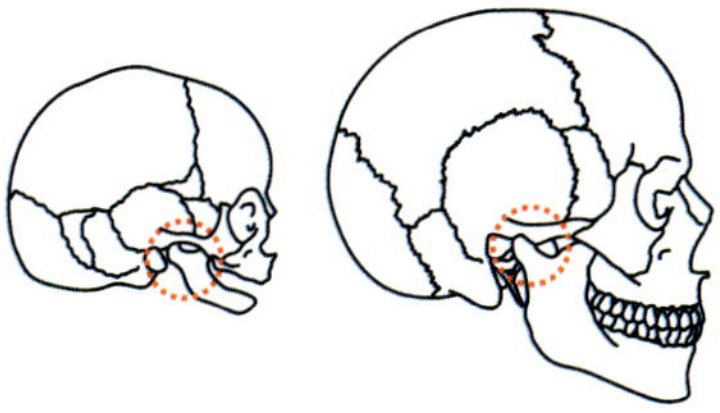

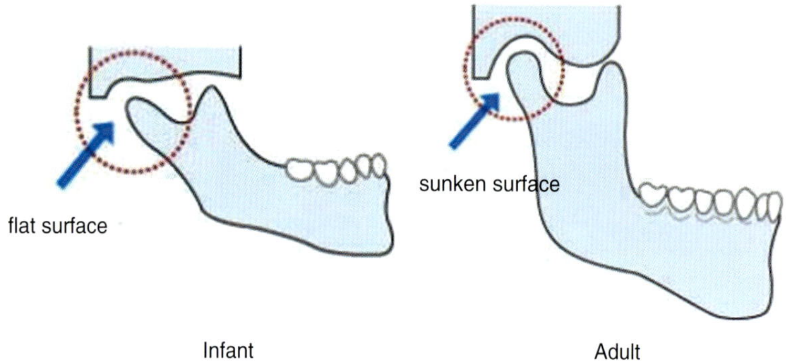

Infant's temporomandibular(jaw) joint has a flat surface which enables the free movement of the lower jaw. Whereas adults have mortar and pestle like bumpy joints which prohibits the free forward movement of the lower jaw.

Infants less than a year old can move the lower jaw freely and easily. And because infants only have front teeth, they tend to stick out their lower jaw every time something is appeared within their reach. However, parents should not permit their infants to stick out their lower jaws out of habit. Such bad habits could lead to excessive growth of the lower jaw, resulting in a baby to eventually have a long and tilted lower jaw later on.

It is too early to determine whether the infant will have a long and tilted lower jaw or not in the future before the baby reaches about the age of three.

G. Artificial Deformation of Bone Structure

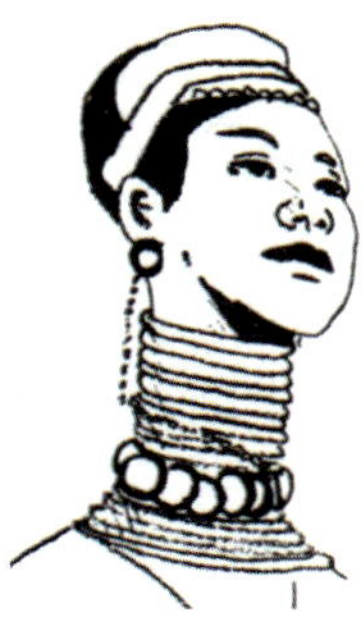

Beauty in Padung region in Miyanma. They think it a yardstick for a beauty who wears lots of metal rings on their necks as many as possible. The rings worn on the neck were removed in their entirety, she can not control her neck.

H. Head Deformation of Incan People

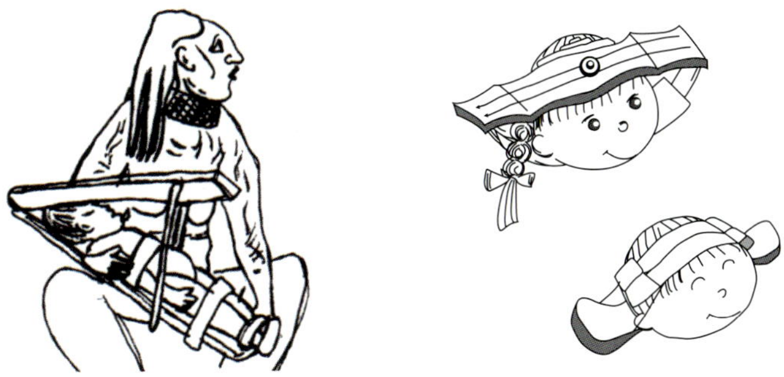

There are various methods for shaping a child's head. One of American natives named Nooksack inserts the infant's head between the wooden plates in order to deform the head shape intentionally. They think this bizarre shape of skull seems to be very brave and strong.

Professions of the Incas were hereditary. Under any circumstances, in order to identify social status they had, head shapes were intentionally modified differently. For example, a king's head was changed tetragon, warrior triangle, farmer rounded- shape etc.

Head deformations usually are carried out just after births and continued for several years until the desired head shape is attained, or the child does not want to wear wooden frame. It is not so painful as expected.

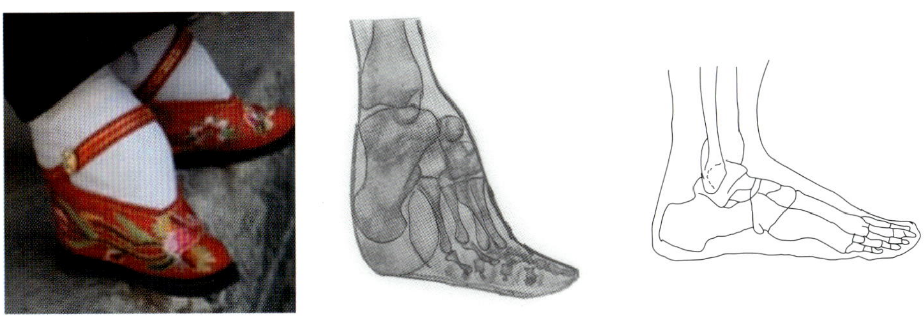

From the ancient times, Chinese women's small feet are barometer of a beauty. So Chinese woman forced to wear small leather shoes from the earlier ages in order not to grow their feet normally. Length of feet didn't reach 10 centimeters (left end photo). Warped foot bone caused by bound feet(center). Right end photo shows normal foot bone.

23. Treatment of Mandibular Prognathism

A. Regular Check-ups

B. Cephalocaudal Gradient of Growth in Human Body

C. Chin Cap

D. Utilization of Chin Cap

E. Treatment Effect

F. Face Mask

G. Treatment by Face Mask

H. Extraction

I. Growth Spurt for Girls

J. Growth Spurt for Boys

K. Utilization of Growth Spurt

L. Functional Orthopedic Appliance

A. Regular Check-ups

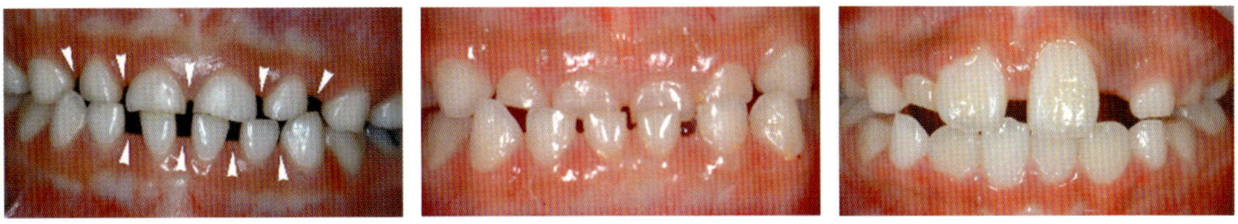

Left figure shows normally aligned teeth of a child. In case of middle figure, the upper front teeth are completely locked inside the lower front teeth, which shows strong sign of long and tilted lower jaw in the future if left untreated early. Right end figure shows an intermediate result of early treatment for the patient of middle figure.

The main cause of long and tilted lower jaw is either the lack of growth in the upper jaw or excessive growth of the lower jaw. In the case of such jaws, front teeth of the upper jaw tilt outward, while the front teeth of the lower jaw tilt inward. Such type of jaws can be diagnosed at the age of about three.

If the infant's one or two front teeth of the lower jaw are somewhat tilted forward despite the normal upper and lower jaw structure, this symptom might be cured spontaneously without any treatment. These infants should have regular check-ups by orthodontists.

If the front teeth of the upper jaw are locked completely inside the front teeth of the lower jaw, early treatment is necessary since the growth of the upper jaw inevitably will be impeded.

B. Cephalocaudal Gradient of Growth in Human Body

The growth rate of the human body tends to increase where the organs or bones are located far away from the head(cephalocaudal gradient). For example, legs grow longer than arms. Likewise, lower jaw, being further away from the head, generally grows more and later than the upper jaw, which is closer to the head. ("cephalo" is a combining form denoting relationship to the head, and "cauda" to tail.)

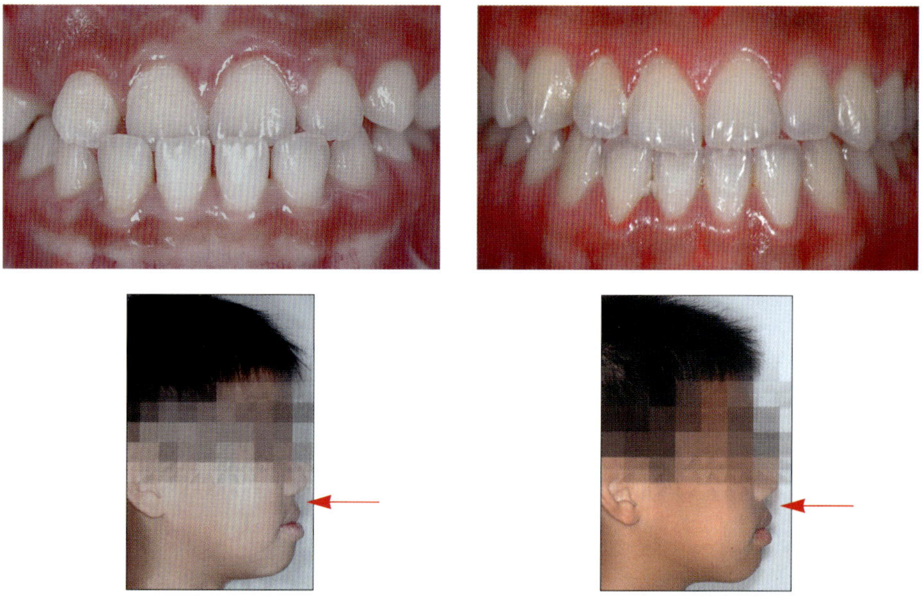

Profile changed after treatment. Shape of upper sunken lip disappeared.

If a child's lower jaw seems to be positioned little bit outward, or if the region between the nose and the upper lip is sunk, it can be said that the child’s lower jaw has higher possibilities of excessive growth, thus enabling the child to have a long and tilted lower jaw later on.

C. Chin Cap

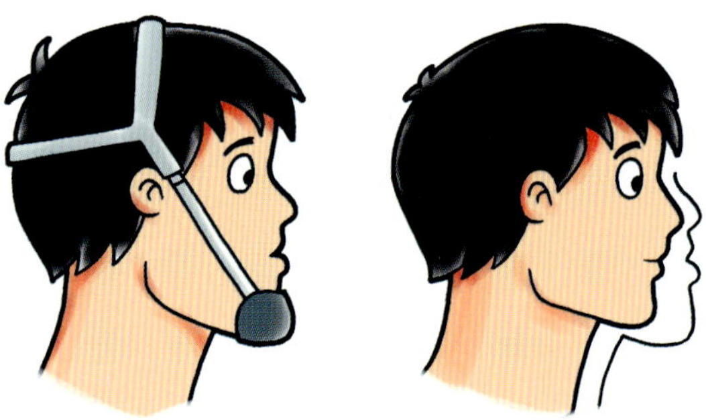

If a long and tilted lower jaw is formed by the excessive growth of the lower jaw, the growth rate of the lower jaw must be suppressed during growth period. For the treatment of this type, the usage of orthodontic appliance called chin cap is required. But, cooperation of the patient is needed, especially in the case of children patients. Patients who are around five to six years old can be expected to cooperate with such treatment.

Chin caps are required to be applied for 13~14 hours (including the time when patients are asleep). After five or six months to around a year, the long and tilted lower jaw will be completely cured. In some cases, additional orthodontic appliance are applied along with chin cap.

D. Utilization of the Chin Cap

Purpose:

To suppress the excessive growth of the lower jaw.

Hours to be used:

If possible, it is recommended that patients wear the chin cap all day long. It must be worn more than 14 hours a day. Chin caps should be removed when having a meal, brushing the teeth, doing sports activities, or taking a bath.

How to keep it clean:

Chin caps often cause rashes to the skin. Therefore, it should be covered with soft cloth on the bottom of a chin cap. Also, when patients are sweating, baby powder should be applied on the bottom of the chin cap. Apply soap to clean the cloth from the dirt.

E. Treatment Effect

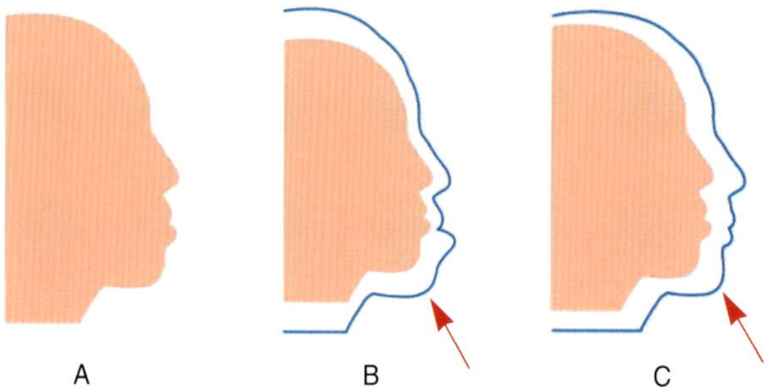

A. Before treatment
B. Unfaithful wearer of chin cap
C. Faithful wearer

F. Face Mask

If the long and tilted lower jaw is formed by poor growth of the upper jaw, rather than excessive growth of the lower jaw, a face mask can be used to promote the growth of the upper jaw.

This treatment is the most effective for children in the 6 to 8-year-old age group, thus the timing is very important.

Similar methods of treatment can be applied in cases of cleft lip and palate patient as well. This is so because the growth of upper jaw of cleft lip and palate patient is severely impeded.

G. Treatment by Face Mask

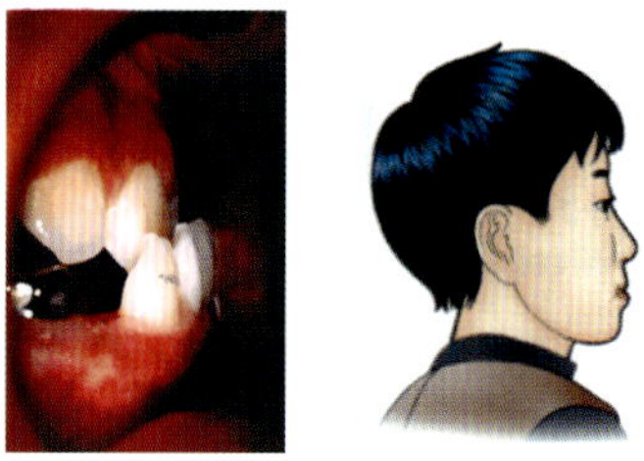

Before treatment of a child with an anterior crossbite

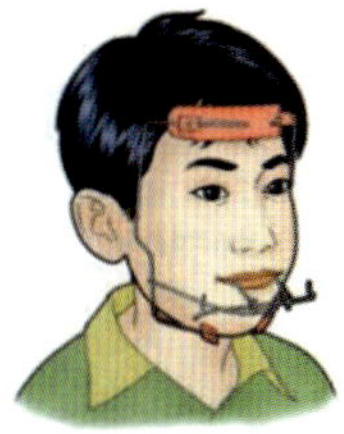

With a face mask on

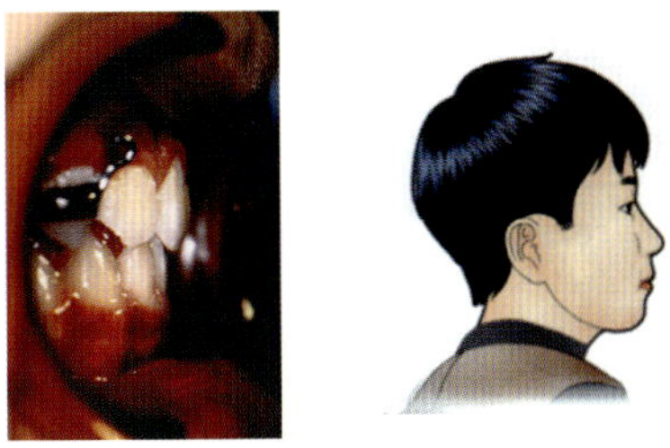

After treatment

H. Extraction

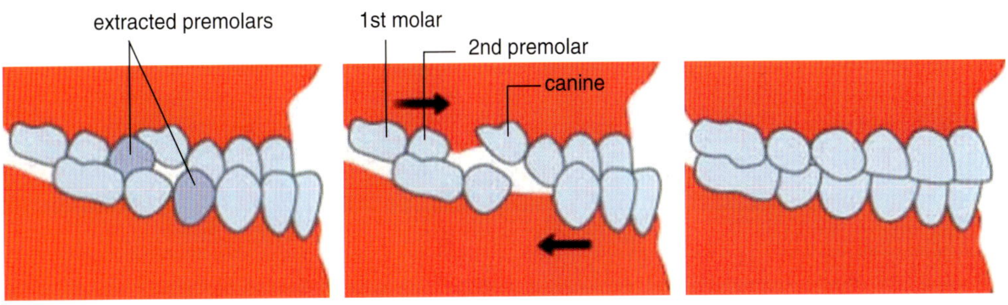

The upper and lower teeth are set in opposite ways(cross bite). Four premolars of upper and lower jaw are extracted, and the upper back teeth (premolars and molars) are shifted forward and the six front teeth(anterior teeth) on the lower jaw are pushed backward. Normal teeth alignment is attained after treatment.

Nowadays, orthodontists tend to select surgery instead of premolar extraction therapy in the case of long and tilted lower jaw. Because extraction of four premolars requires reasonably long period of occlusion adjustment, furthermore, overall facial esthetics are compromised by the strong appearance of the chin. Only surgery accompanied by orthodontic treatment must improve the overall facial esthetics as the patient desire(refer to photos on page 128).

I. Growth Spurt for Girls

The peak velocity for physical growth coincides with development of sexual characteristics such as noticeable breast development, darker and wide pubic hair, appearing hair in armpits. Menstruation begins 1 to 1.5 years after sexual characteristics appeared. By the time of the onset of menstruation, the girl's growth spurt is all but complete.

J. Growth Spurt for Boys

The characteristics of sexual maturation in boys increase in body fat. At this time boys may appear obese and somewhat awkward physically, and also the scrotum begins to increase and changes its color darker.

Growth spurt begins 1 year after the sexual maturation has appeared. At this time redistribution and relative decrease in fat, pubic hair begins to appear, and growth of the penis begins.

Growth spurt begins later and extended over a longer period about 5 years compared with 3.5 years for girls.

K. Utilization of Growth Spurts

Temporary improvement of the long and tilted lower jaw during growth period does not mean that the treatment is complete and stable. A person goes through stages of growth spurts twice in a lifetime, which usually coincides with the sudden increase in height.

This phenomenon usually occurs around the time he/she enters elementary school and again at the time of graduation of elementary school.

The biggest growth spurt occurs during the second growth spurt period when the puberty and adolescence begins, and the biggest growth spurt occurs on the average nearly 2 years earlier in girls than in boys.

At this time, the lower jaw will grow longer excessively, thus it may ruin the previous treatment. Therefore, a chin cap must be worn until the patient reaches the end of growth spurt.

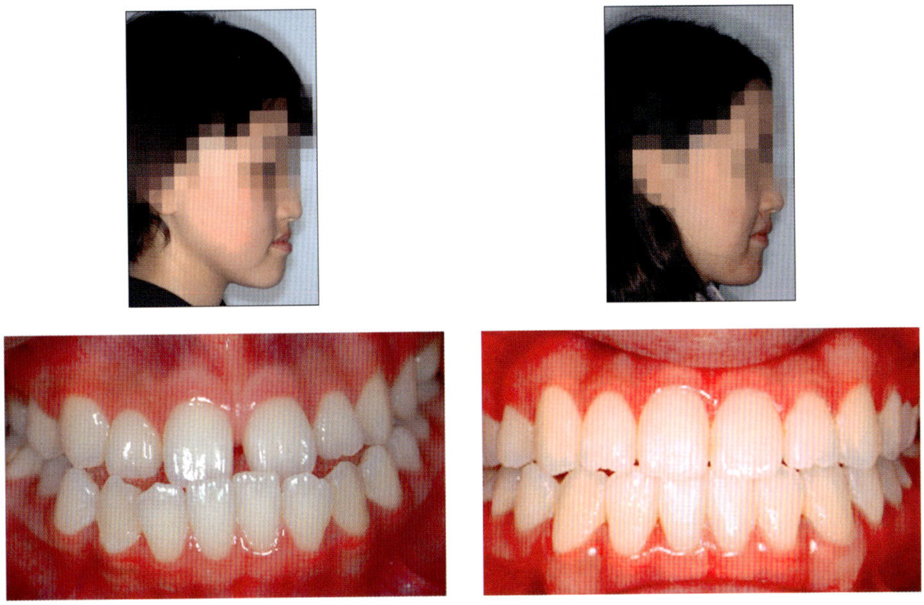

Before and after treatment of long and tilted lower jaw tendencies during her growth spurt.
Chin cap is worn during her night sleep until the end of growth spurt period.

L. Functional Orthopedic Appliance

If the lower jaw has developed more than the upper jaw, the upper teeth are caged in by the lower teeth. If the patient is a child who is in his growing period, an orthodontic appliance which enables the upper jaw to grow more than the lower jaw is used. This appliance is a kind of functional orthopedic appliance which uses muscle function and the most typical appliance is called "Twinblock".

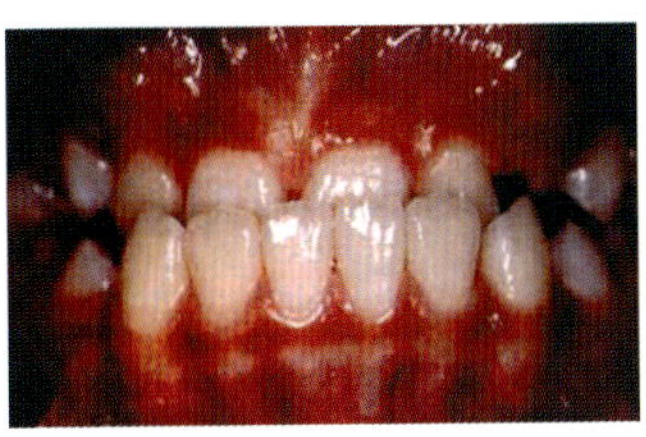

before treatment

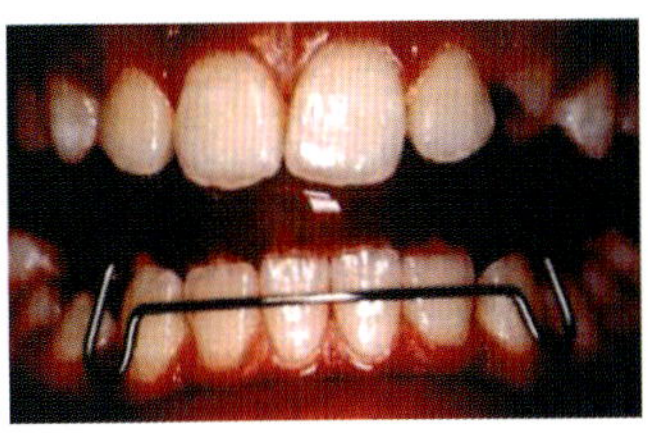

wearing the Twinblock

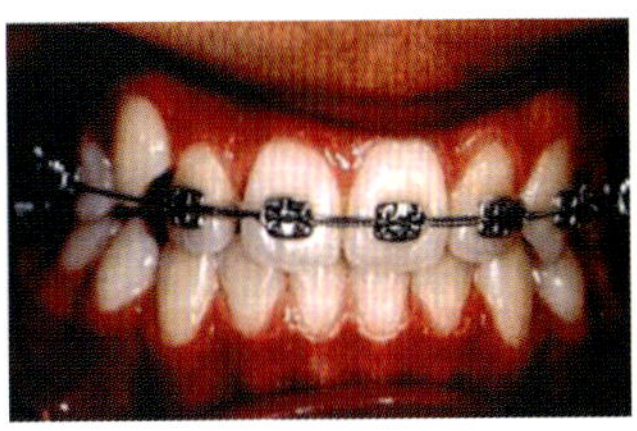

wearing brackets

Through the use of Twinblock, growth of the two jaws were controlled normally. However, the teeth were not completely aligned in spite of Twinblock treatment, so brackets were used for short-term period.

24. Orthognathic(Plastic) Surgery

Definition:

Surgical treatment of structural abnormalities of the jaws and resulting in facial harmonies.

A. What does it mean?

B. Combination Therapy with Orthodontics and Surgery

C. Slightly Protruded Lower Chin

D. Facial Asymmetry

E. Underdeveloped Chin

F. Underdeveloped Lower Jaw

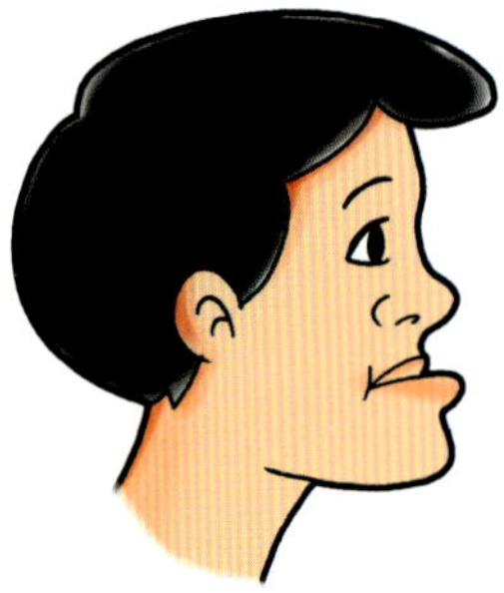

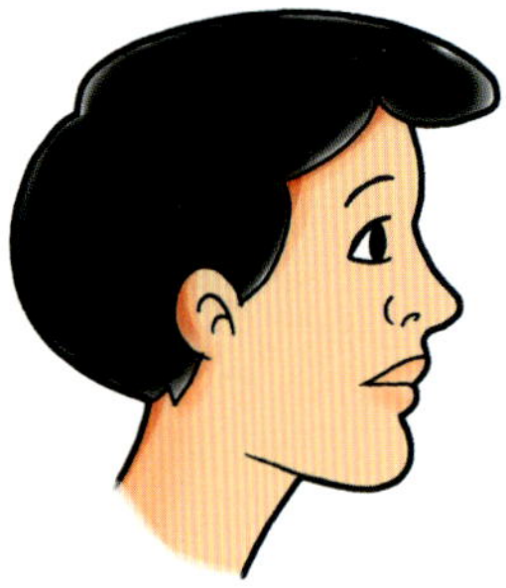

A. What does it mean?

There are many expressions used to describe a person's facial appearance such as "having a long face like a horse", or "having lips like cherries". Each person has his own facial characteristics such as big jaws, slanted eyes, hooked nose, or dimpled face etc. We can all agree that the person's face looks somewhat odd if some parts of face such as nose, mouth, eyes are out of balance.

A certain person's eyes, nose, and mouth may look beautiful if you look at each part carefully, but looking at them all together as a whole, it may somehow seem odd. This may be the case of a lady who does not look pretty because her facial features are out of balance.

On the other hand, a person's eyes, nose, and mouth may not look beautiful one by one, but when viewed as a whole, this person's face may be appealing.

The shape of the face and the balance of the ears, eyes, mouth, and nose are the factors that decide facial beauty. If there is an imbalance among parts of the face, it is natural for the face to look unbalanced.

The shape of the face can be an idiosyncrasy, so as long as there is no particular imbalance, subtle makeup and a certain hair style can help to obtain a better image of oneself.

However, if the lower jaw is abnormally long, or if the upper jaw is severely protruded, making the face look somewhat unbalanced, then it may be impossible to obtain ideal results through orthodontic treatment alone. Unbalanced face may cause the person to develop an inferiority complex.

In this case, it is recommended that the person receives a combination therapy with orthodontics and oral surgery to regain self-confidence. This procedure is called "corrective surgical treatment", or "orthognathic surgery(Greek word, *ortho* means straighten, *gnathos* jaw)".

B. Combination Therapy with Orthodontics and Surgery

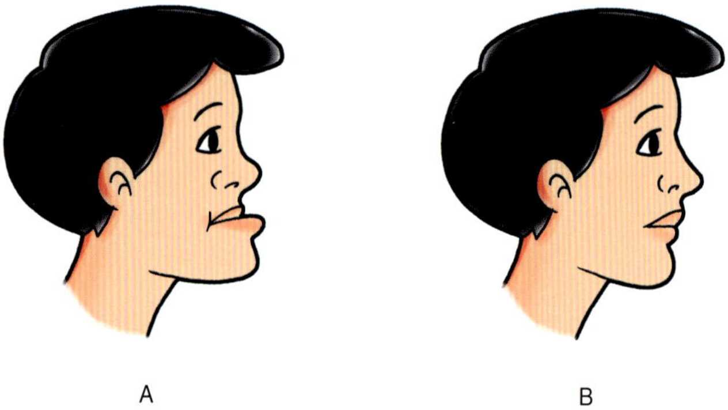

A: Before treatment
B: After combination therapy with orthodontics and oral surgery

C. Slightly Protruded Lower Chin

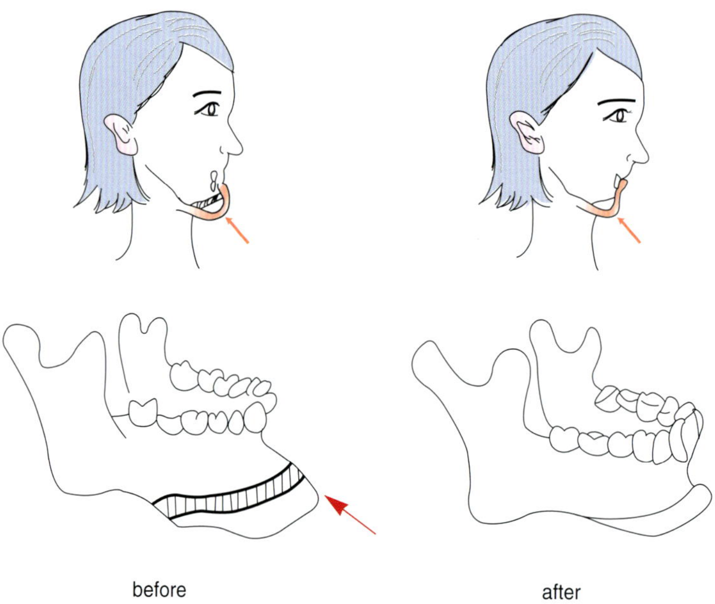

If the relationship between the upper and lower jaw is normal and only the chin is slightly protruded, it can be treated only by shaving off the chin.

But if chin is severely protruded as shown above illustration, lower jaw is horizontally cut off and pushed back. The chin is split into 3 layers, and then middle layer is discarded. The lower layer is pushed back.

D. Facial asymmetry

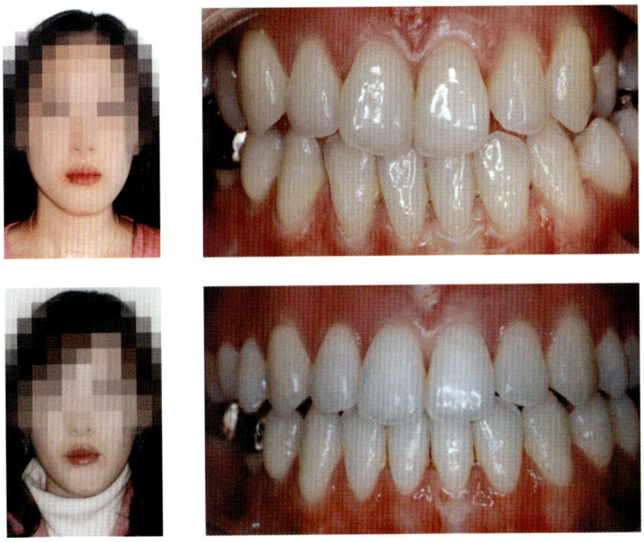

The asymmetric face was corrected only by orthodontic treatment.

E. Underdeveloped Chin

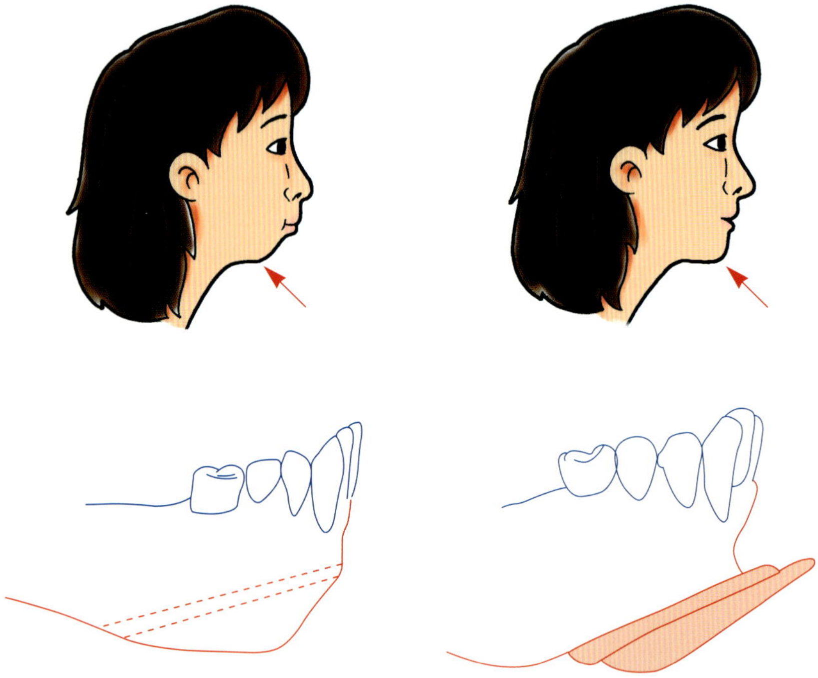

before treatment after treatment

Complete, favorable teeth alignment is attained through orthodontic treatment, but the patient looks awkward because of a small-sized chin. In this circumstance, facial esthetics can be improved through surgery. The chin was split into three layers and the lower layer was pulled out and elongated.

F. Underdeveloped Lower Jaw

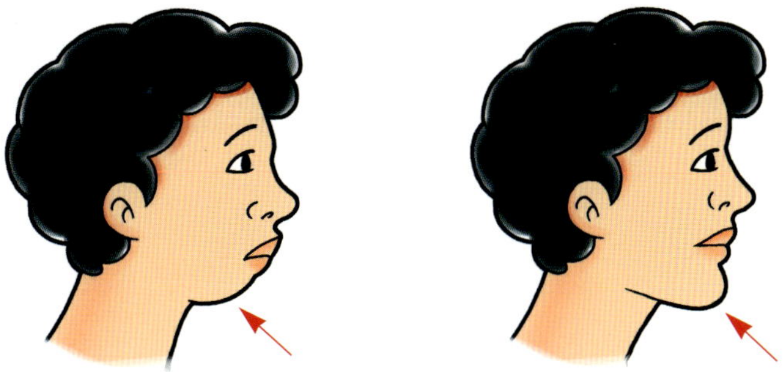

before treatment after treatment

A person with a small lower jaw and chin somehow portrays the image that he/she lacks will power. Even the neckline may look awkward, which may make the person appear foolish. On top of that, when the person passes age of 30, the neckline and chin get thicker, and the drooping of the skin may become noticeable. Thus, the person looks much older than someone with a fairly normal chin.

In this case lower jaw was cut off vertically to stretch outward. Of course the excision is made inside the mouth so there are no visible scars.

After combination therapy the line between the chin and the neck is noticeably improved giving a much better appearance.

VI. Combination Therapy

25. Combination Therapy for Long and Tilted Lower Jaw (Orthodontics and Orthognathic Surgery)

A. Outline of Orthognathic Surgery

B. Orthodontic Treatment before Orthognathic Surgery

C. Orthognathic Surgery

D. Orthodontic Treatment after Orthognathic Surgery

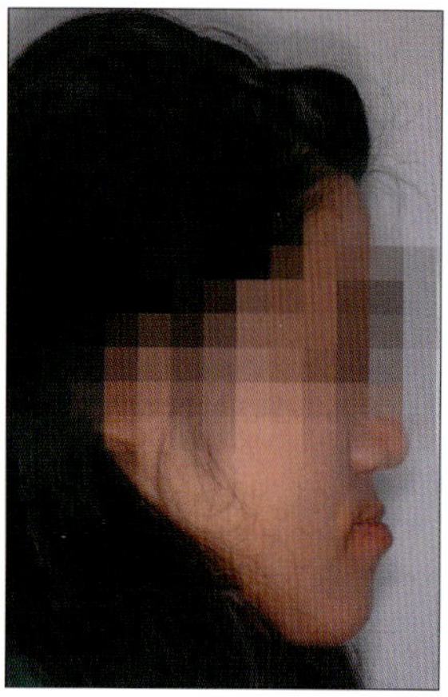

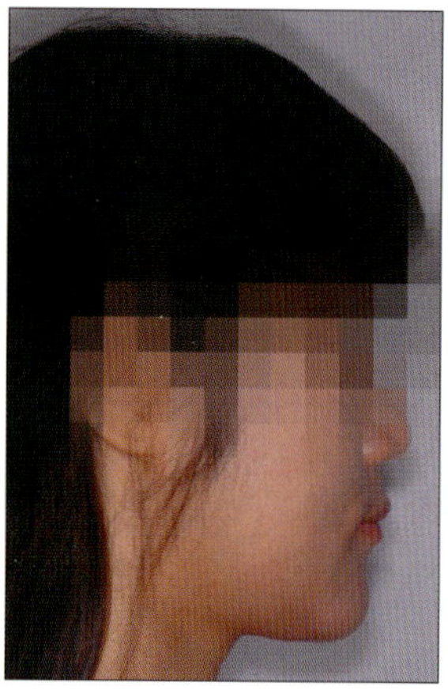

A. Outline of Orthognathic Surgery

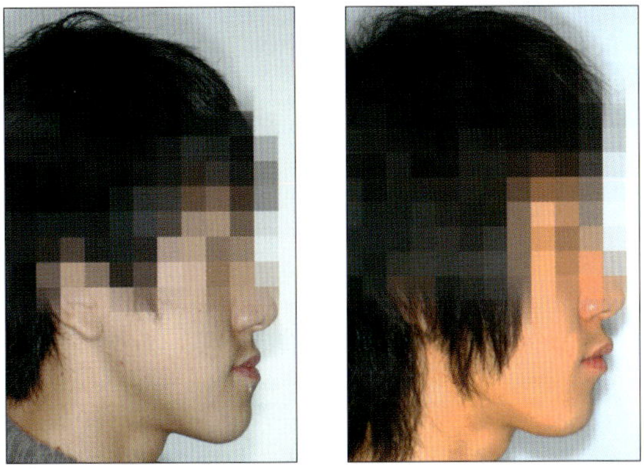

Although the teeth alignment has improved only by orthodontic treatment(left), the external shape of lower jaw has not changed at all. In a case like this, surgery must be accompanied by an orthodontic treatment. Right photo shows orthodontic/surgical outcome. The Oral Surgeon cut off the lower jaw and pushed the front part of lower jaw backward.

If a person wishes to correct long and tilted lower jaw at the age of 17 or 18, then it can be corrected only by orthodontic treatment with extraction in 2 years. But, since the ugly external appearance of the lower jaw is being left alone while the only teeth alignment is being corrected.

In this case, in spite of orthodontic treatment, there will not be much difference in the appearance, and even the good aligned teeth would look unnatural.

Because of the rapid advances in the field of oral surgery, a wide range of treatment possibilities have opened recently. So the number of adults who wishes to have better facial appearances are increasing day by day.

Also in the case of adults, who cannot treat long and tilted lower jaw with only orthodontic treatment, combination therapy must be performed.

You must first consult your orthodontist, discuss the possibilities of how the teeth alignment and facial profile will change after combination therapy, and then you can begin orthodontic treatment before surgery.

The surgery is performed under general anesthesia within the mouth, therefore, no external scars will be left. The patient will receive orthodontic treatment again after surgery.

With orthodontic treatment accompanied by oral surgery, even the most severe case can be treated nowadays.

B. Orthodontic Treatment before Orthognathic Surgery

Combination therapy is performed in 3 stages; before surgery, surgery itself, and orthodontic treatment after surgery for fine correction of the teeth between the upper and lower jaw(occlusion).

A person with an abnormal skeletal feature also has teeth alignment that goes along with it. If the surgery is performed without orthodontic treatment, it will be difficult to obtain the accurate occlusion when the skeletal feature returns to normal after the surgery.

For this reason, it is necessary to obtain normal teeth alignment beforehand. Orthodontic treatment before surgery takes about a year. And its procedure is almost the same as the usual orthodontic treatment.

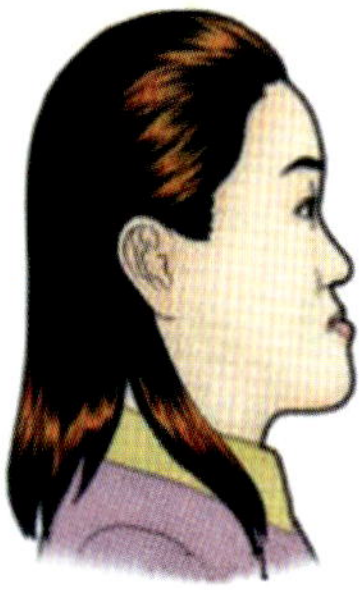

A

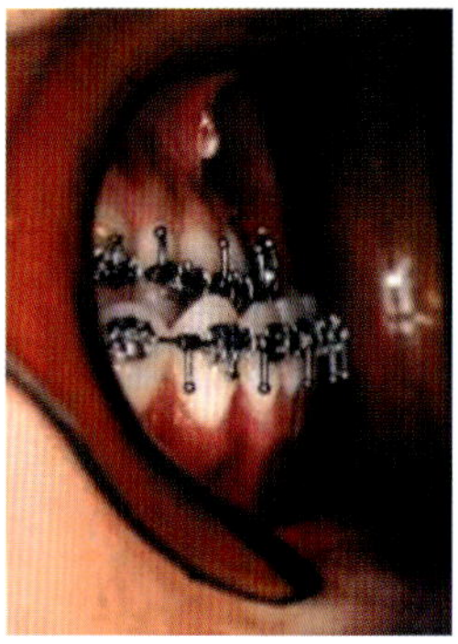

B

A: profile before treatment
B: orthodontic treatment before orthognathic surgery

C. Orthognathic Surgery

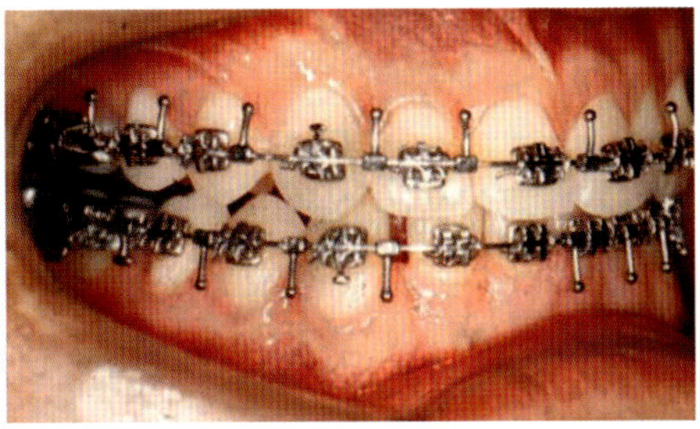

just after surgery

When normal teeth alignment has been obtained through orthodontic treatment before surgery, the orthodontist will confer with the oral surgeon about the facial changes after surgery based on the data gathered from x-rays, photos, and study model of the patient's natural teeth in position(dentition).

Most of the procedures are done in the mouth, so the external scars will be invisible. The lower jaw is cut off to obtain normal relationship between the upper and lower jaw, then the fixation will be done for 4~6 weeks to heal completely. Until the bones heal completely, the patient will take soft food.

D. Orthodontic Treatment after Orthognathic Surgery

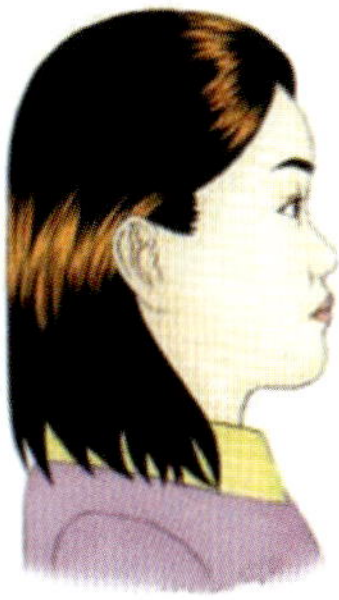

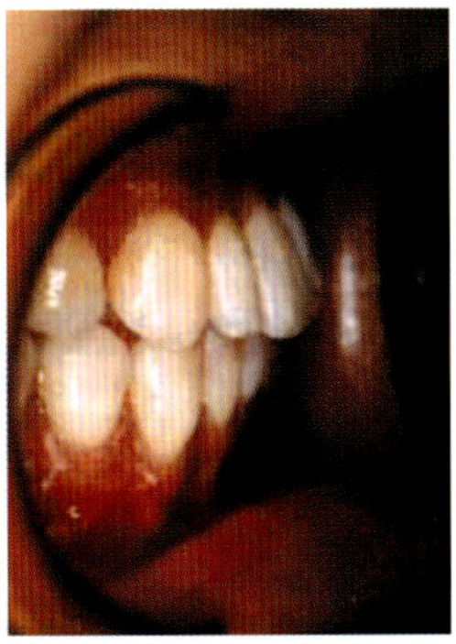

orthodontic / orthognathic surgery outcome

After surgery, physical therapy for intentional opening and closing the mouth is performed.

When the skeletal position is altered through surgery, there will be slight changes in the muscles and their functions to compensate for new position. Only when the facial muscles are adapted to a new position completely, the normal relationship between the upper and lower jaw will be kept stable.

Furthermore, to prevent and compensate relapse due to surgery, orthodontic treatment is performed in the same manner as it was done before surgery to obtain an accurate position of the upper and lower teeth. This procedure will also take about a year.

26. Corticotomy

A. Treatment Limitations for Adult Orthodontic Patients

As the life span increases recently, the number of adults who want to change their facial appearance and correct their teeth alignment are increasing continuously. Adults want to have their complications to be solved in a short period of time.

There are many difficulties in adult orthodontic treatment compared to young age. The adult bone is very thick, and reduced blood supply results in reduction of overall metabolic activity. Therefore, in case of adult patient even though the same movement occurs, it is slower and it takes longer for the teeth to take their new stable positions after treatment.

Adults are much slower in adapting to new environments compared to children. As a result, there are limits to adult orthodontic treatment.

In adults, there are also cases where the root of the teeth become resorbed after treatment.

Growth modification treatment as in adolescence also can not be chosen, because the period for the control of growth and development has already passed in adult's patients(refer to Functional Orthopedic Appliance Page on 158).

B. New Paradigm Appeared for Adult's Orthodontic Patients.

Before the introduction of "corticotomy" in the Orthodontics, it is generally accepted that controlling the overall alignment of the teeth through comprehensive orthodontic treatment is possible up to the twenties. Naturally, after the age of 30, only partial orthodontic treatments are usually performed until recent years.

To meet these patients' demand for short treatment time and overcoming the age limitations, "corticotomy" incorporates into the adult orthodontic treatment procedure.

Corticotomy procedures are not brand new method and have now been in practice for more than a hundred years ago.

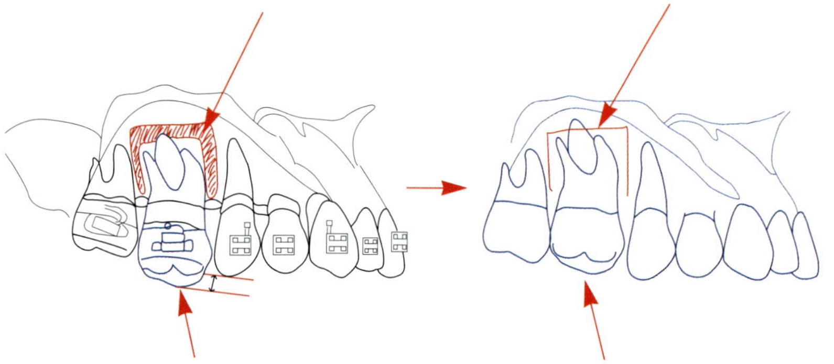

Superficial hard layer of bone is called cortical bone. A fissure is made through the cortical bone(hatched zone) that surrounds a tooth so that the tooth is embedded within a block of bone that is connected to adjacent blocks through only the inner side of bone(bone marrow). This method allows much faster tooth movement, thereby making it possible to shorten the treatment time.

27. Cleft Lip and Palate

A. What Is Cleft Lip and Palate?

B. New Born Infant

C. Initial Surgery

D. Orthodontic Treatment Begins.

E. Orthodontic Treatment Finished

A. What is Cleft Lip and Palate?

When we say “cleft lip and palate”, we usually refer to a congenital condition where the upper lip and palate is torn out, and is one of the most common congenital facial malformations. Approximately 1 in 700 children are born with this misfortune. It is also referred to as "harelip" because it resembles the lips of a hare.

The earliest recorded case of successful repair of a cleft lip appears to be around AD 390 in China.

With the developments in plastic surgery, if proper treatment is received, there should be no functional problems in daily life. It is also not a hereditary abnormality.

B. New Born Infant

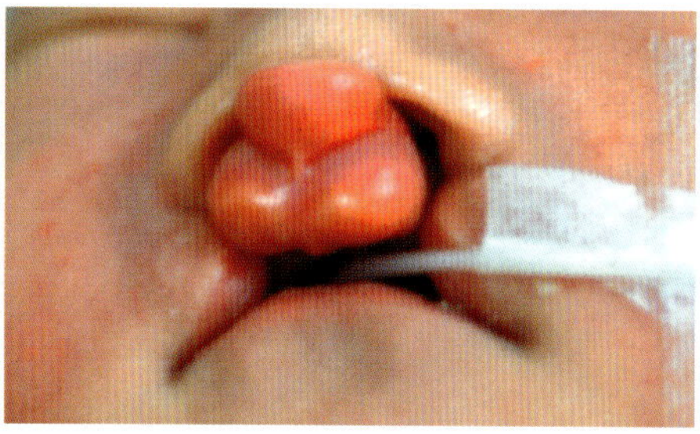

Just after birth

(by courtesy of Professor Jung-Keun, Lee, Affiliated Dental Hospital, Ajou University, Suwon, Korea)

This infant was born with a complete bilateral cleft lip and palate. Because the upper lip and palate separated, the child cannot suck milk and the appearance is quite unattractive. If a simple appliance called “Hotz plate” is inserted for milking, the infant will be able to grow normally.

C. Initial Surgery

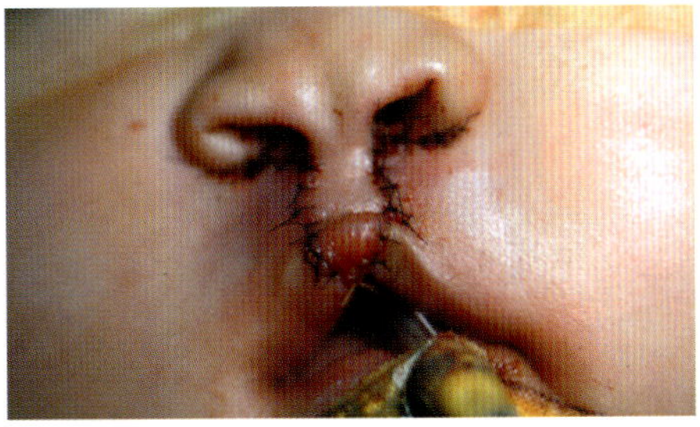

Initial surgery

(by courtesy of Professor Jung-Keun, Lee, Affiliated Dental Hospital, Ajou University, Suwon, Korea)

The separated upper lip makes it difficult to pronounce words properly and the separated palate makes the child susceptible to respiratory disease such as flu, tonsillitis, sinusitis.

Therefore, when the child reaches a certain weight, surgery will be performed to close the separated lip and palate. It leaves a scar and the nose becomes lopsided, so plastic surgery for reshaping the nose will be done afterwards.

D. Orthodontic Treatment Begins

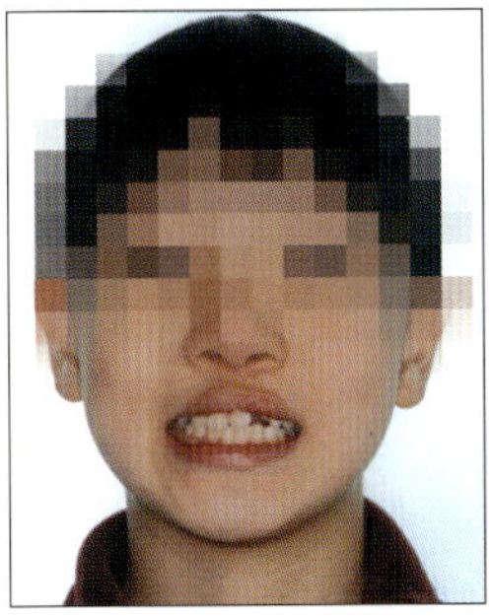

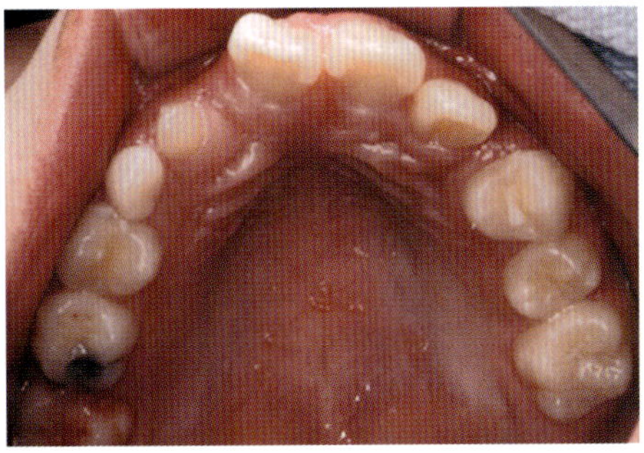

After the lip and palate are closed through surgery, it will create a hard scar issue as it heals. Because this scar tissue is very tough, the upper jaw will not be able to grow normally. Furthermore the bone surrounding region of the affected teeth does not grow properly, and the teeth alignment becomes crooked.

Also, cleft lip and palate patients frequently have several missing teeth, so orthodontic treatment is performed after the first surgery.

E. Orthodontic Treatment Finished

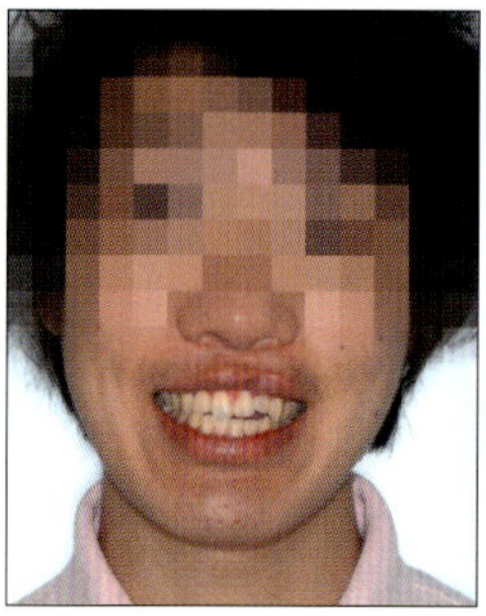

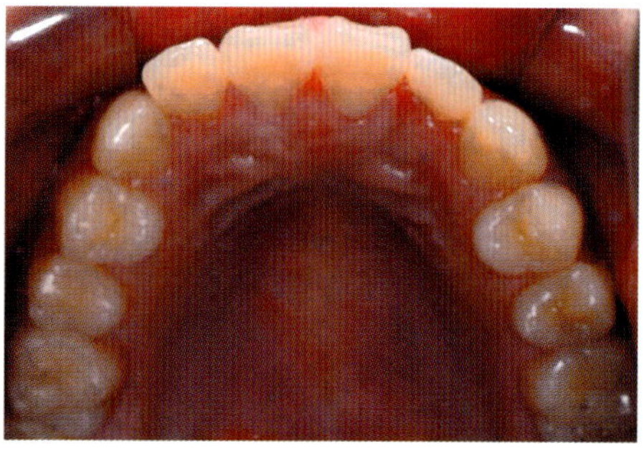

Orthodontic treatment has been completed in several stages. The teeth alignment is good and now there is no difference from the appearance of a normal person.

Through plastic surgery, the scar on the lip has been disappeared and the nose has been restored, leaving no functional and psychological problems in daily life.

VII. Orthodontic Treatment for the other Purposes

28. Orthodontic Treatment in Case of Accidents

A. Shortened Crown Caused by Fracture

B. Elongation by Orthodontic Appliance

C. Completion of Treatment

D. After Treatment

E. Elongation by Orthodontic Treatment and Crown Reshaping

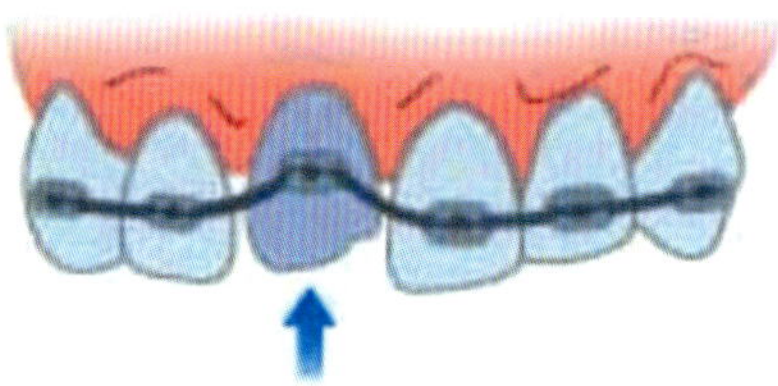

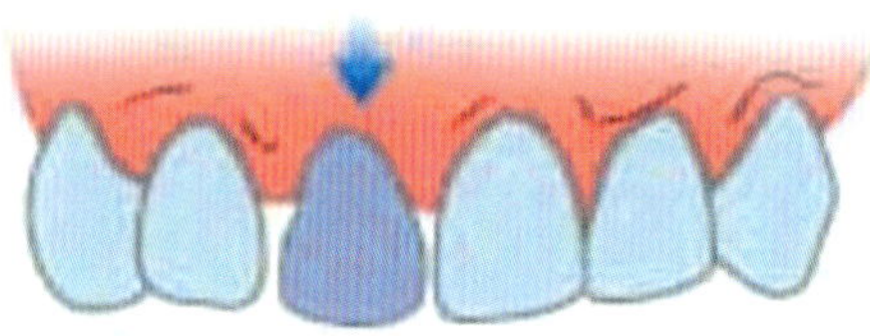

A. Shortened Crown Caused by Fracture

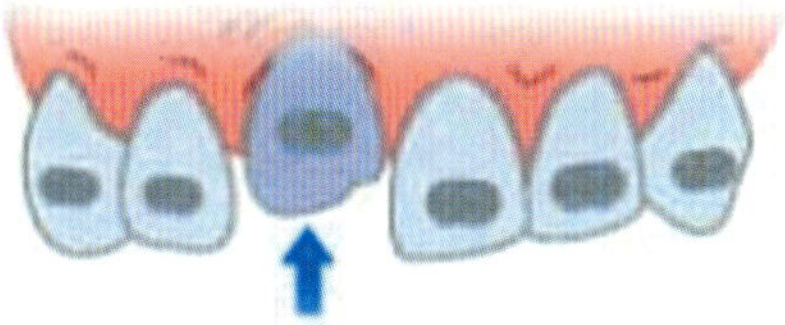
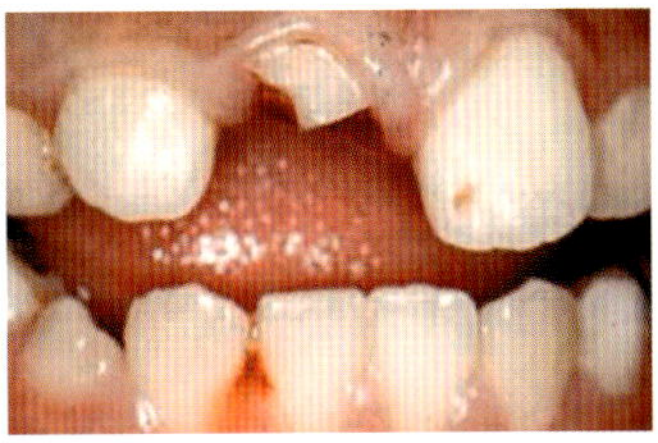

If a tooth has been broken through some kind of sports activity, accident or trauma, it is difficult to make a normal artificial crown because of its shortened length of tooth crown. Therefore, orthodontic treatment is performed to bring the tooth to the level of its adjacent teeth, then the crown is placed.

B. Elongation by Orthodontic Appliance

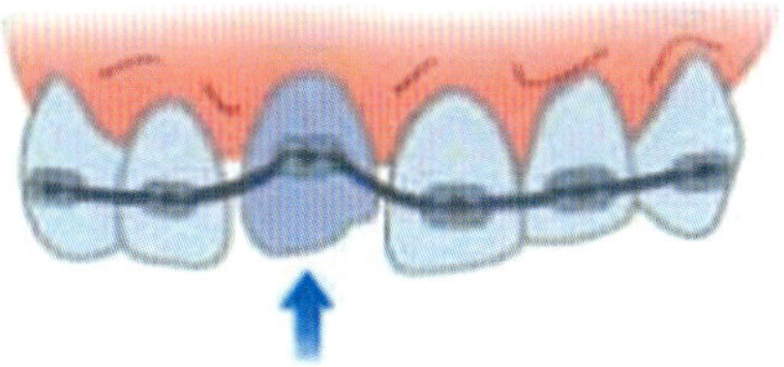
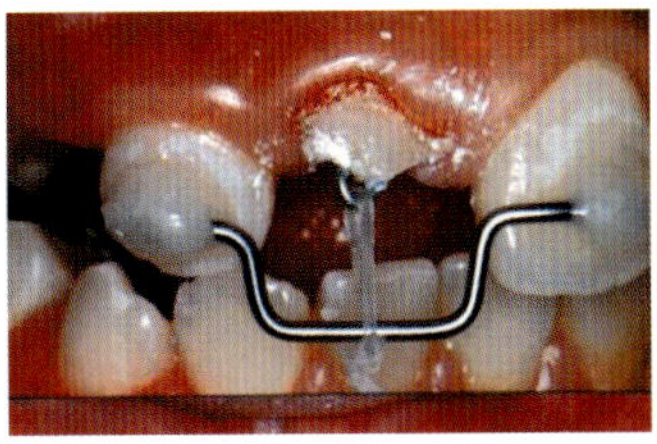

Orthodontic treatment is done in order to elongate the tooth until reaching the same level of adjacent teeth.

C. Completion of Treatment

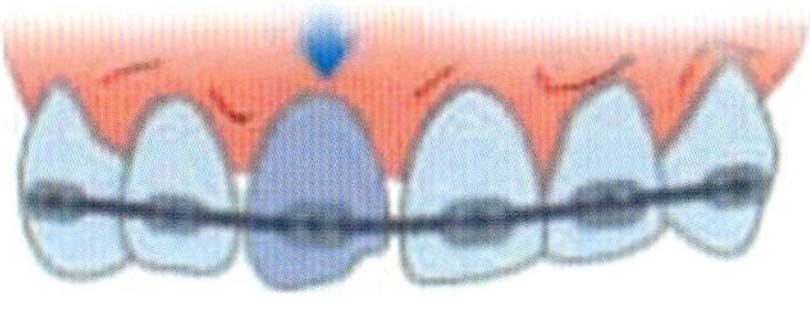
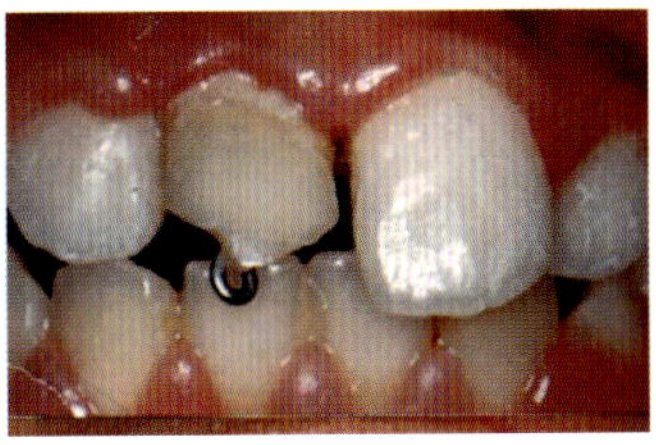

The length of broken tooth reaches almost the same level as adjacent ones.

D. After Treatment

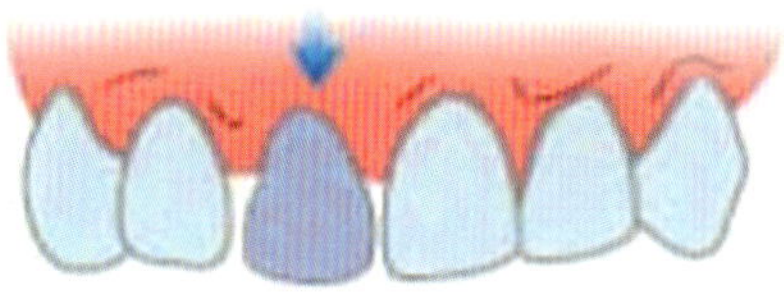
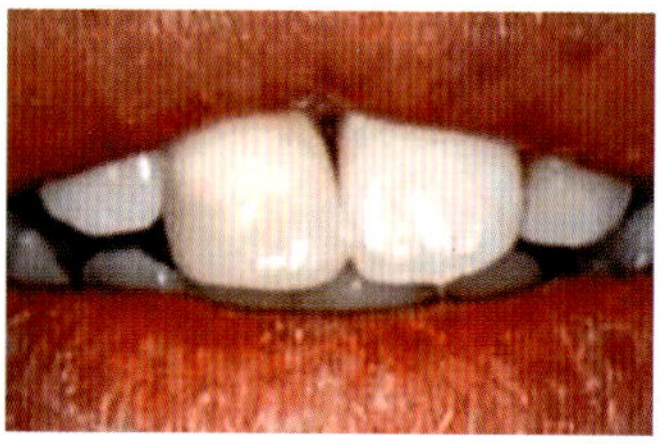

Normal shape and appearance attained after treatment.

E. Elongation by Orthodontic Treatment and Crown Reshaping

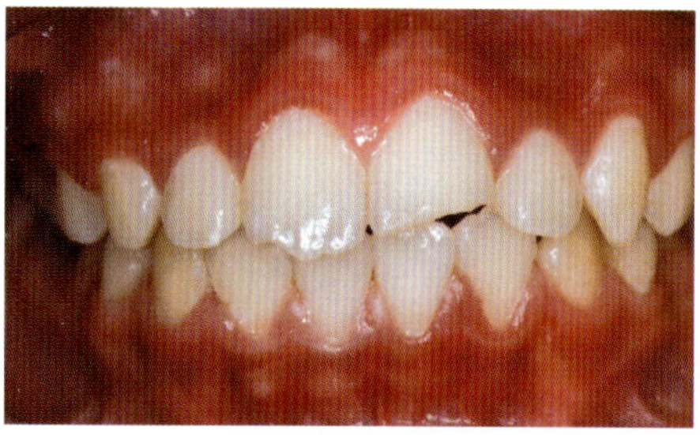
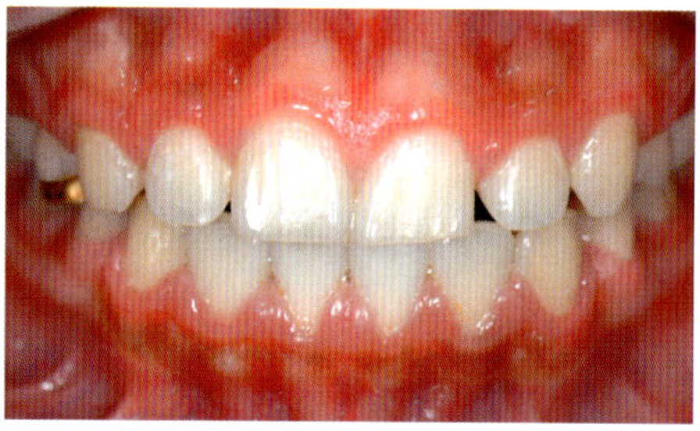

The crown of upper front teeth is shortened by trauma. It is elongated by orthodontic treatment to the level of its adjacent teeth, and then reshaped by tooth-colored resin.

29. Orthodontic Treatment for Temporomandibular (Jaw) Joint

A. Normal Function of Temporomandibular(Jaw) Joint

B. Effect of Teeth Alignment on Temporpmandibular(Jaw) Joint

C. Temporomandibular(Jaw) Joint Problems

D. Splint Therapy

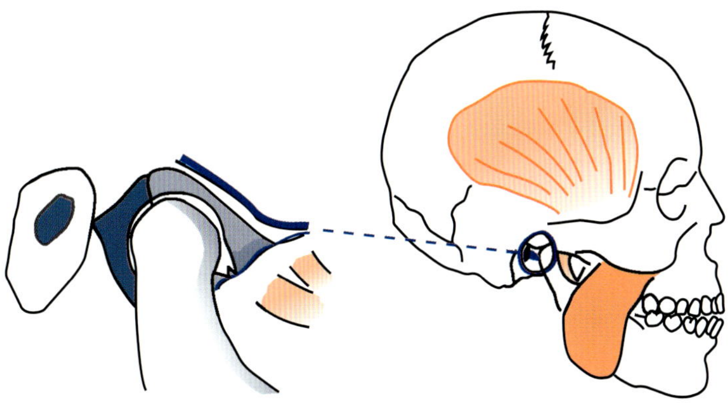

A. Normal Function of Temporomandibular(Jaw) Joint

In order for temporomandibular(jaw) joint to maintain its normal function, the muscles around the face and neck, and inter-digitation between upper and lower teeth (occlusion) must keep harmony.

B. Effect of Teeth Alignment on Temporpmandibular(Jaw) Joint

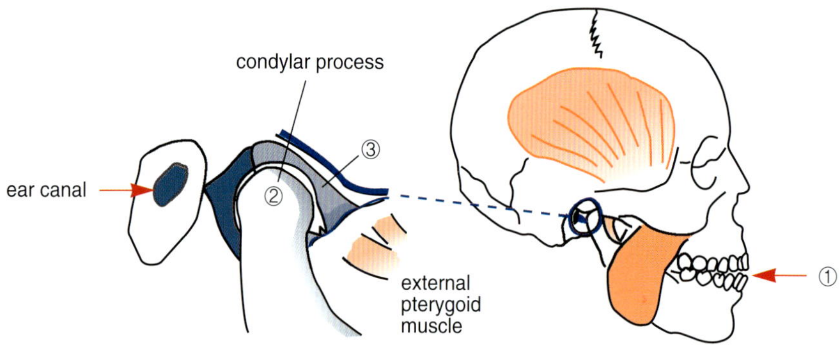

1. If the upper front teeth is tilted inward, the lower jaw is likely to subject to backward pressure whenever closing the mouth.
2. Head of jaw joint saddled in backward.
3. Articular disk is pushed out and then temporomandibular(Jaw) joint problems ensues.

C. Temporomandibular(jaw) Joint Problems

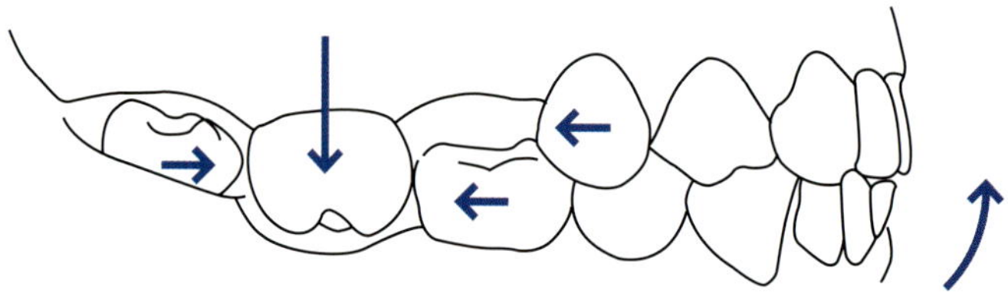

Poorly aligned teeth and stressful daily life can cause temporomandibular(jaw) joint problem. People with a poorly aligned teeth normally seem to have no problems in daily lives, but facial muscles are excessively used while chewing food since they cannot chew as effectively as normal persons. Thus, it can bring stress to the jaw joints.

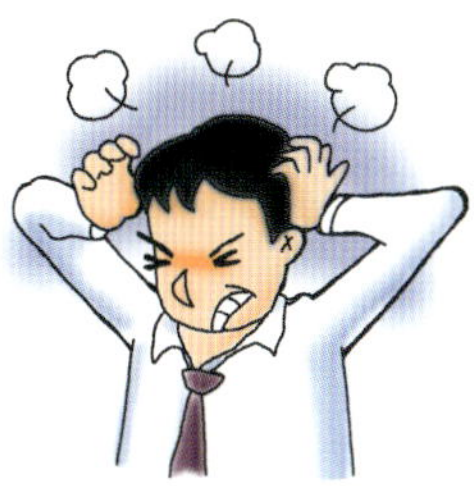

stress

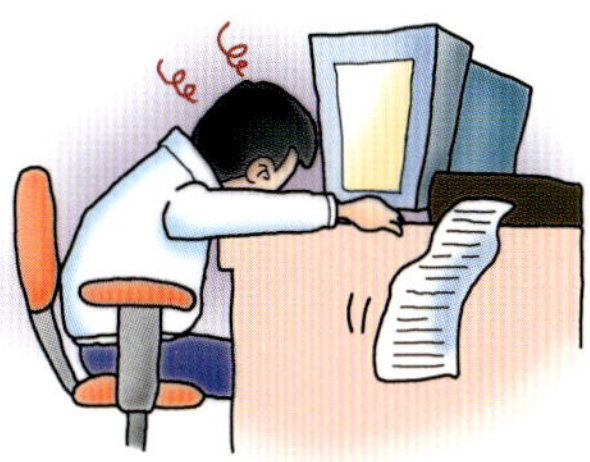

fatigue

When persons are continuously exposed to stressful situations or mental fatigue, then unconsciously clenches the mouth during the day work and subsequently grinds the teeth severely in their night sleep.

This will bring stress to the temporomandibular joints causing symptoms like headache, eye fatigue, shoulder pain, or noise in the ear when opening and closing the mouth.

This is called "temporomandibular joint syndrome" and orthodontic treatment can be selected to alleviate these symptoms.

D. Splint Therapy

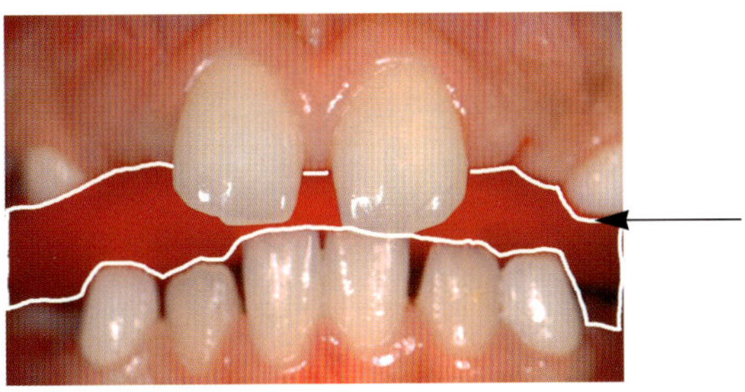

The relationship between the upper and lower teeth are not in balance, it causes problems in function of temporomandibular joint and severe pain during opening and closing the mouth. An appliance called a splint is used to alleviate the pain and tension on jaw joint.

30. Orthodontic Treatment in Adults

A. Collapsed Extraction Space

B. Keeping Parallelism

C. Pretreatment for Implant

D. Your Own Teeth Is the Best.

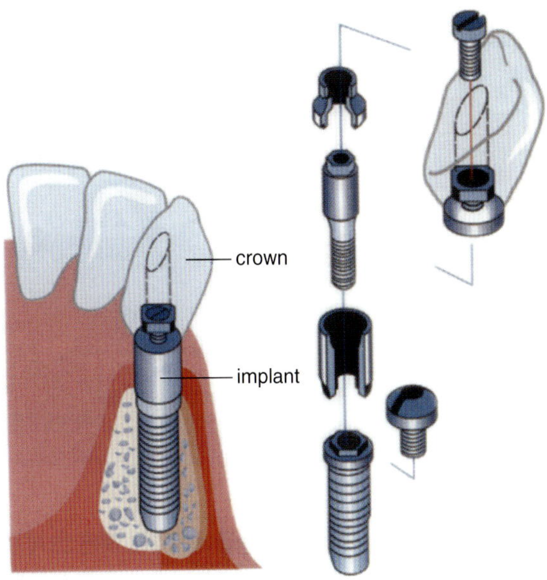

A. Collapsed Extraction Space

Children and adolescents are not the only ages who receive orthodontic treatment. Adults in their 40s and 50s can receive orthodontic treatment as a pre-treatment for crown and bridge(prosthesis) or to obtain a balance in the chewing force applied to the teeth.

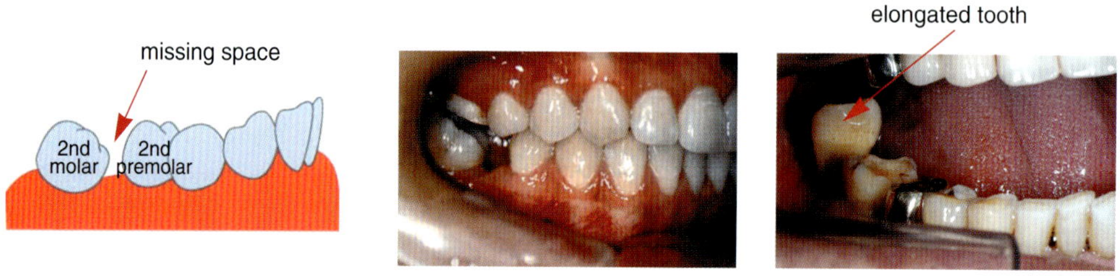

If the space where the tooth had been extracted is left untreated for a long time, the adjacent teeth will tip each other and the opposite teeth will be elongated.

In severe cases shown in right end photo, the molar on the lower jaw will grow into the space where the molar tooth had been extracted on the upper jaw. This makes it difficult to obtain an ideal crown and bridge(prosthetic) treatment.

B. Keeping Parallelism

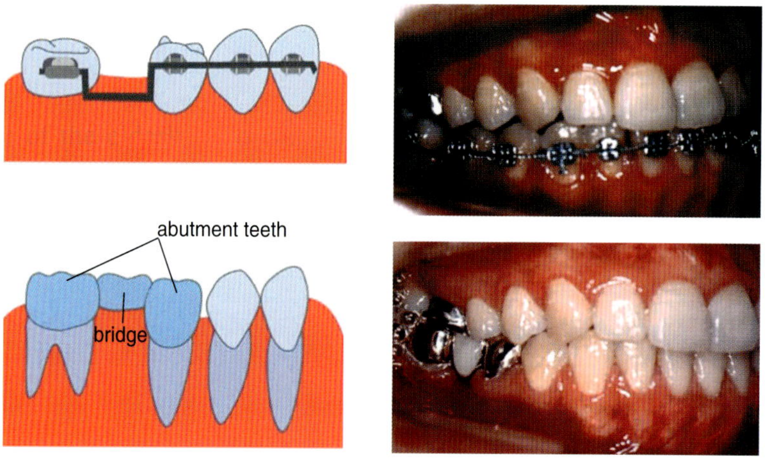

After uprighting the abutment teeth, the crown and bridge is placed.

In prosthetic treatment(crown and bridge), it is most important to maintain parallelism of the adjacent teeth where the crown and bridge, or artificial tooth such as implant may be placed.

In the treatment of crown and bridge, both end teeth are called abutment teeth. In order to insert the prosthesis(artificial teeth) correctly, these abutment teeth must be uprighted to their normal position to obtain parallelism.

C. Pretreatment for Implant

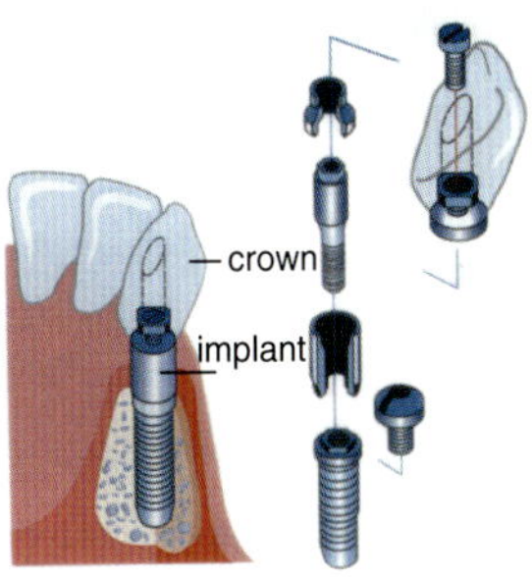

implant currently used

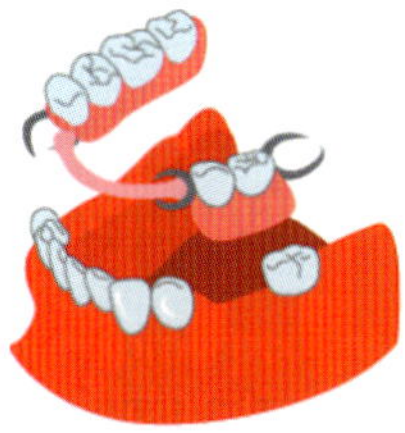

Until recently, this kind of partial denture is widely used when several teeth are missed.

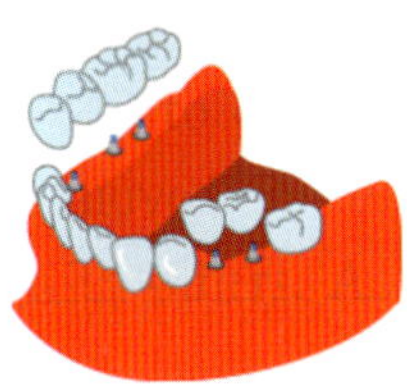

Currently, implant therapy is firstly considered in case of missing several teeth like in this illustrations.

Sometimes orthodontic treatment is necessary for perfectly functioniong implant. In order to plant the opitimal-sized implant correctly and keep the good function, the most important thing is to attain the sufficient space before implant placement.

D. Your Own Teeth Is the Best

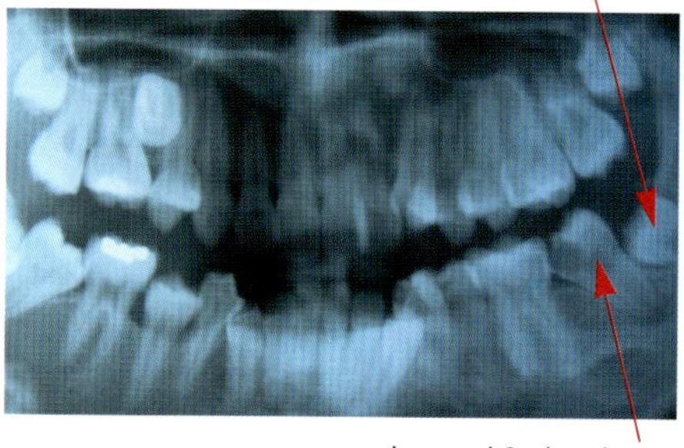

A

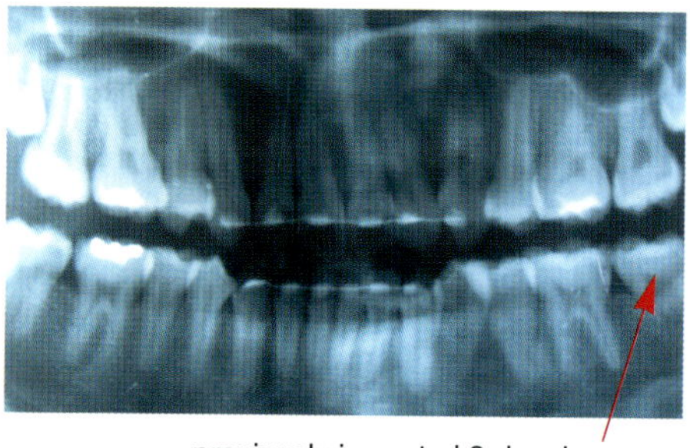

B

Right second molar was removed because of severely decayed(A). Impacted wisdom tooth(third molar) was moved forward by orthodontic treatment, finally reached normal function.

Orthodontic treatment is always better than crown and bridge or partial denture treatment. The only advantage of crown and bridge treatment is that it takes less time. Teeth are seemingly very hard, but because they have living cells, nerves, and blood vessels, they can sense the nature, temperature, and texture of food. No matter how effective an artificial tooth is, it can never match a function of natural tooth.

Recently some dental hospitals or other dental care institutions establish tooth bank, and have begun to collect and store the individual's wisdom teeth(3rd molar) for future use.

VIII. Kinds of Orthodontic Appliances and Tooth Brushing

31. Orthodontic Appliances

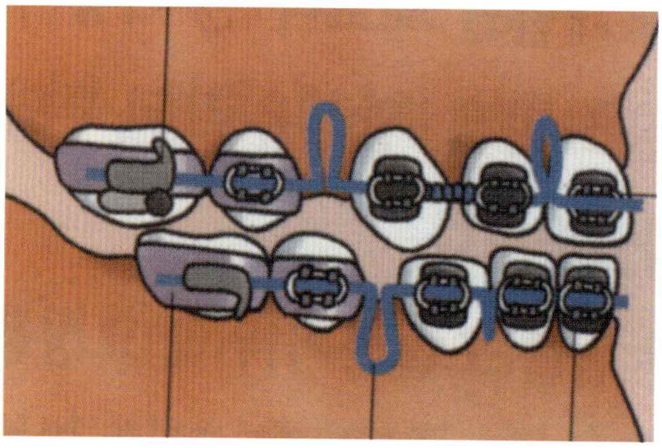

A. Two Kinds of Orthodontic Appliance

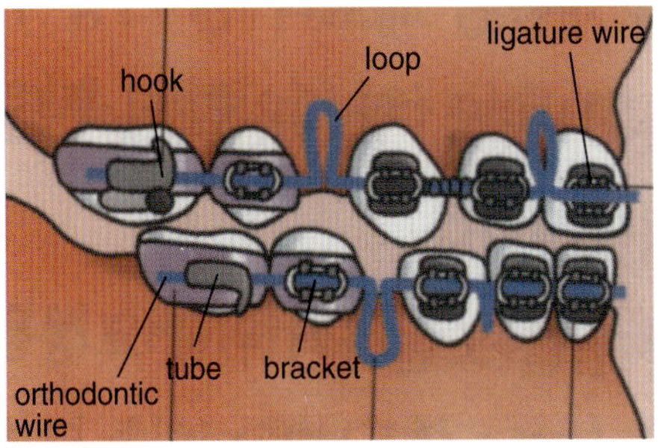

fixed type appliance

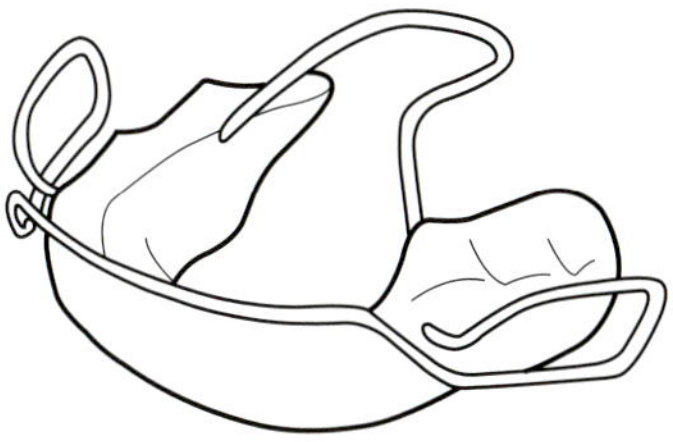

removable type appliance

Largely there are two kinds of orthodontic appliances. One is the fixed type with metallic or ceramic pieces called bracket that are bonded on the teeth and the other is the removable type. Every patient prefers to wear simply looking removable types like the ones that can be removed whenever they want to or wear only in their night sleep.

The effects of each appliances are very different, so a patient cannot choose which appliances to use. The orthodontist will choose the appliance that is simple and will not interfere with daily life such as eating, talking and sports activities. So, the patient should not choose an appliance just for convenience, because this will decrease the effectiveness of treatment, and under circumstances problems can not be solved at all.

B. Visible Labial Metal Bracket

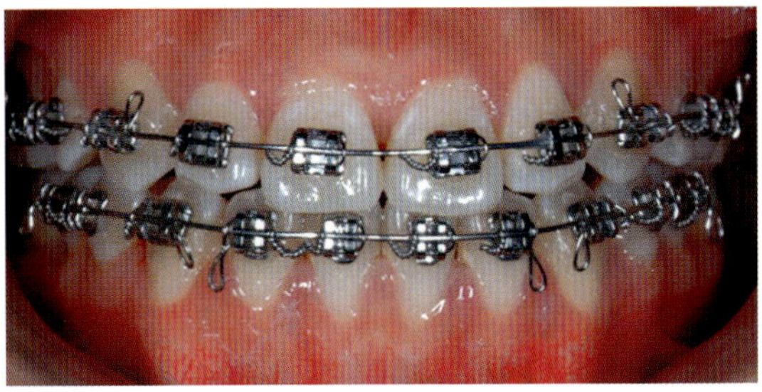

In orthodontic treatment, small hard pieces called brackets are bonded on the tooth surface, and an orthodontic wire is inserted into the bracket slot, and ligate it with a thin wire tightly. Thereafter, teeth start to move to their desirable position.

C. Self-Ligating Bracket

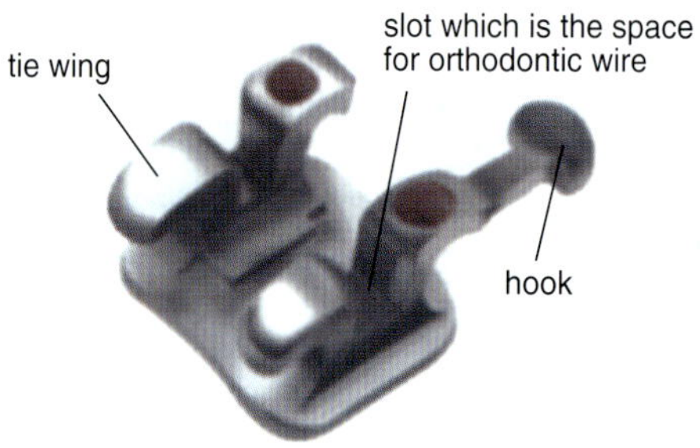

conventionally-ligated bracket

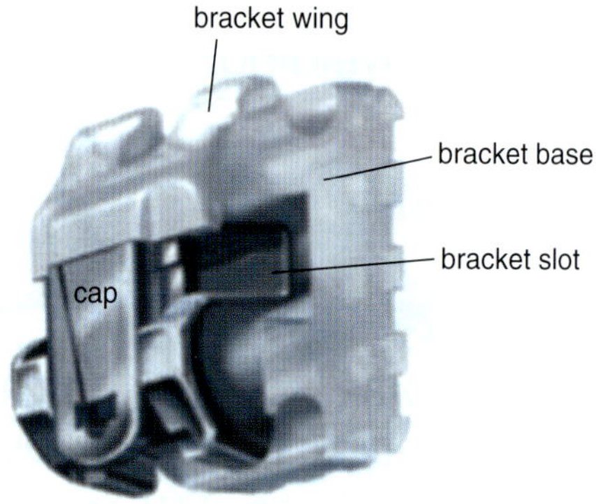

self-ligating bracket

Placing wire ligatures around tie wings on brackets to hold archwire in the bracket slot can be a time-consuming procedure.

Recently brackets which require no ligation are developed and becoming widely spread on the market. It has a cap built into the bracket itself to hold wires in position. Contrary to general thought, it is sometimes very hard to attain precise occlusion in the final step of the treatment.

D. Invisible Lingual Bracket

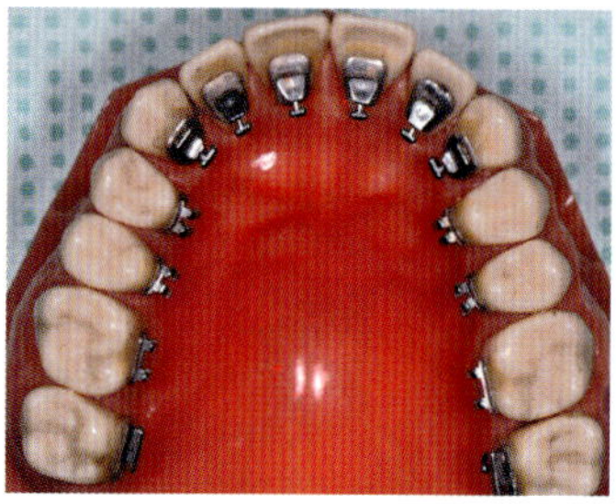

Recently, a lingual orthodontic treatment method of bonding the brackets on the inner side of tooth(so named lingual) has been introduced through the mass media without mentioning its several problems. This caused confusion among many patients.

Since the brackets are bonded and orthodontic wires are inserted into the inside of the mouth, it will be difficult for the patient to talk, chew, and brush thoroughly.

Also since the procedure has to be done inside the small oral cavity, it is also difficult to manipulate the orthodontic wires, so it takes a longer time.

The distance between the brackets is short so it has to be adjusted more frequently, and during each visit, the orthodontic wire almost always has to be completely removed from the mouth in order to adjust.

Thus, it is more difficult, expensive and time-consuming than the usual method. Furthermore, if the occlusion is extremely bad or if a lot of teeth are missing, this method cannot be used.

Less severe bad alignment of teeth can be treated with this current lingual appliance.

E. Clear Bracket

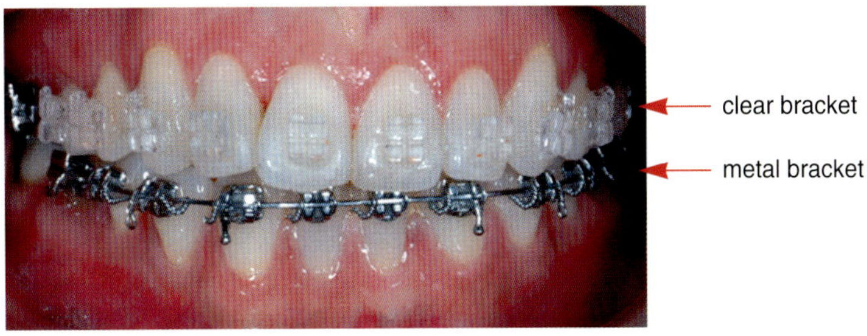

Clear plastic brackets were the first attempt to make metal brackets almost invisible. But this bracket was not durable enough to keep in the mouth, intolerable to bite force, easily discolored, abraded, and broken. The initial failure of clear plastic bracket was one of a major incentive toward the development of lingual bracket.

With the development of ceramic brackets in the late 1980s, the situation changed. The color is very clear, did not discolor and patients appreciated their better esthetic qualities.

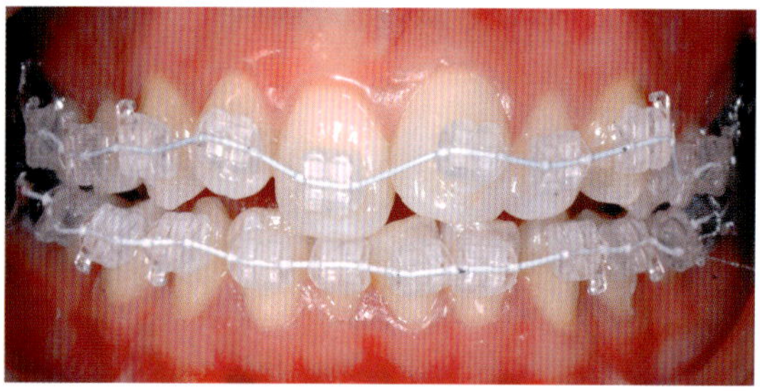

ceramic brackets with tooth-colored glass fiber orthodontic wire

Ceramic brackets are considerably satisfied with the doctor and patient. Furthermore, recently tooth-colored orthodontic wires made by optical glass fiber are on the market. If ceramic brackets are used with this kind of glass fiber wire, orthodontic appliances become almost invisible. As a result, the use of lingual appliances have declined and there are not so many people that really need the lingual brackets any more.

Hoping that other people will not notice that you are receiving orthodontic treatment is unrealistic. Orthodontic treatment has become socially acceptable these days, so there is no reason to hide this fact. Patients' expectations can be met through orthodontic treatment. And if the patients can face other peoples' view with confidence, then it will not matter whether the appliance is showing or not.

F. Occlusal Plate

Among the removable appliance, there is a simple appliance called a "occlusal plate" that is made with plastic and wire. It is frequently used to move one or two teeth that may disturb the teeth alignment in the future if it is left untreated.

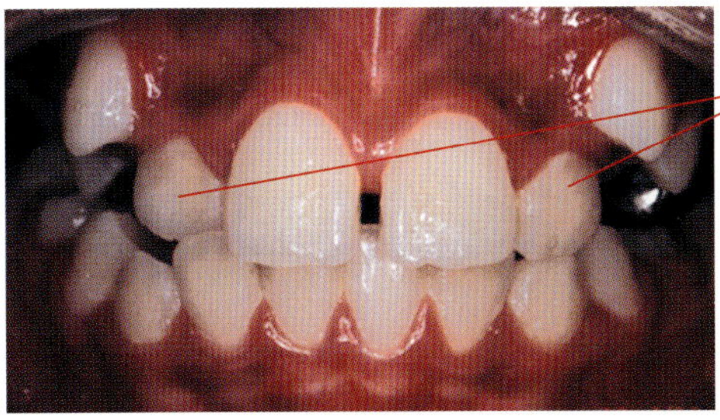

The upper lateral incisors are locked inside the lower incisors(anterior crossbite). The jaw cannot move freely from side to side, so food is chewed only up and down like a rabbit.

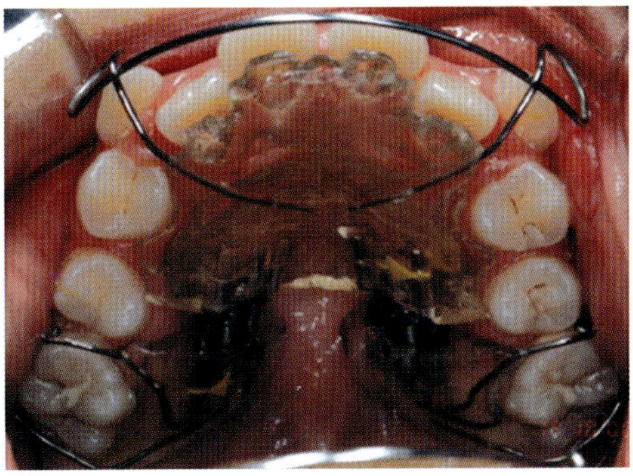

Wearing occlusal plate. Patient can remove and insert it at anytime as he please

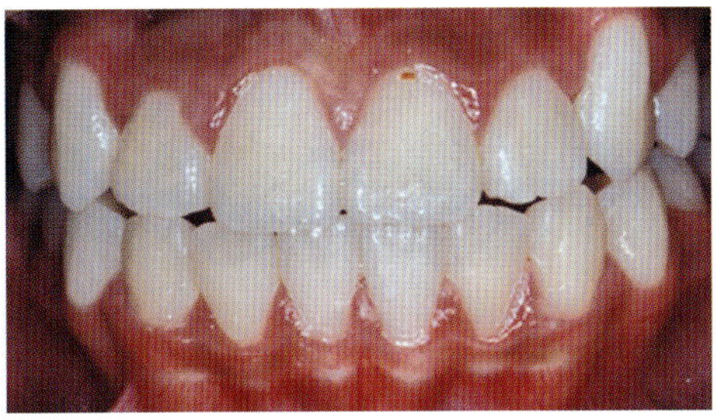

Completion of the treatment in 3 weeks.

G. Functional Orthopedic Appliance

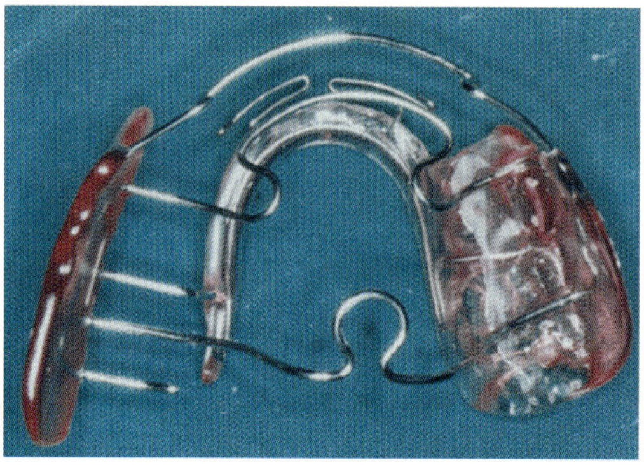

There is another type of removable appliance called the Functional Orthopedic Appliance, which is also made of plastic and wire. This is used to stimulate the growth of jaw bone.

The idea is that forcing the patient's lower jaw to be positioned forward, the growth of lower jaw would be stimulated by controlling the movement of the tongue and the physiological function of the muscles around the region of the head and neck.

Retainers used after the treatment of using the brackets to prevent the teeth from returning to their original state are also one of these appliances. Since these appliances are inserted inside the oral cavity, they are also called the "intraoral appliance".

H. Extraoral Appliance

An appliance worn outside the mouth is called "an extraoral appliance" and because it is exposed to other people, the patient often rejects it.

These appliances are usually connected or used in conjunction with the appliance worn inside the mouth. Most of them are used only for a certain duration of time during the treatment period. They are most often used after school hours and during the night, but in severe cases, they should be worn all day long.

I. Kinds and Usage of Extraoral Appliance

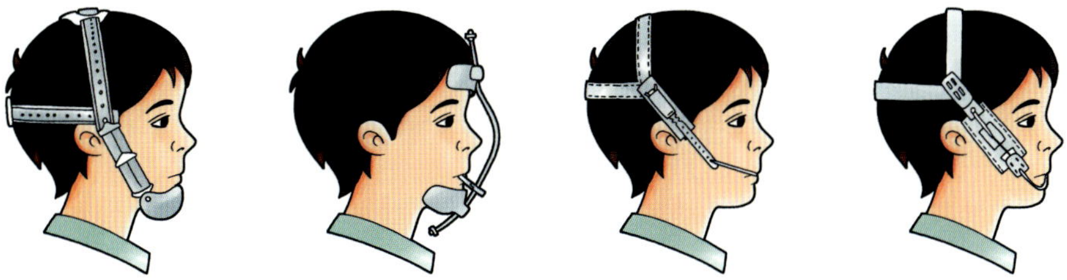

chincap facial mask facebow headgear

Headgear is mainly used for inhibiting the growth of upper jaw in case of the protruded upper jaw. Chin cap is used in case of long and tilted lower jaw for inhibiting the growth of the lower jaw, and a facial mask is used to pull the upper jaw forward.

J. Anchorage in Tooth Movement

Newton's third law of motion says "Two every action, there is always an equal opposite reaction." This principle is applied to orthodontic tooth movement as well.

When forces are applied for the purpose of moving the tooth, there must be greater resistance in opposite directions by several methods. We call this method "anchorage establishment". The anchorage establishment in orthodontic treatment implies resistance to tooth movement.

Anchorage can be obtained by simply binding groups of teeth, using additional appliances or wearing elastics. Extraoral anchorage such as headgear is very effective if complete patient cooperation is obtained. Only when the patient wears this appliance at least 12~14 hours a day, desirable results may be obtained. The more the patient wears this appliance, the better the results will be.

K. Utilization of Mini Pin for Anchorage

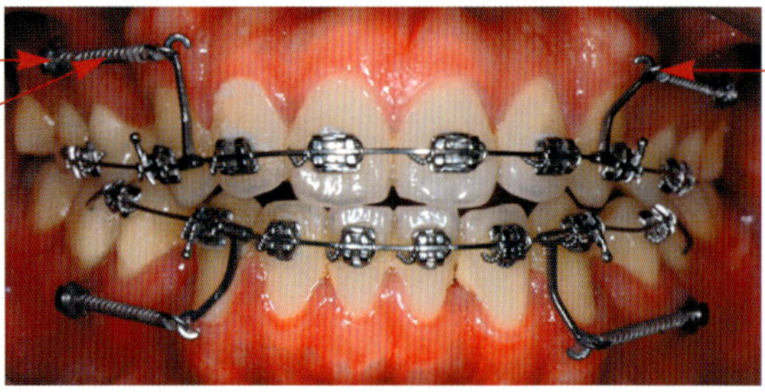

Recently mini pin is widely used for anchorage during orthodontic treatment. Mini pin can replace the visible extraoral appliance such as headgear for tooth movement, and space closure by bringing front teeth backward without any additional appliance can be done easily.

Mini pin can be easily planted into the jaw bone, removed easily as well, and patient's cooperation is not needed. Elastic chain, thread or coil springs can be attached 2~3 weeks after pin planting and it is not so expensive. In addition, it can shorten the treatment period 3~6 months less without patient's cooperation.

L. Invisible Plastic Tooth Aligner

Some kinds of invisible plastic tooth aligner is recently introduced to treat a bad alignment of the teeth. Series of aligners are made on the patient's teeth model, and then wear over the patient teeth. Wearing the aligners step by step will gradually move the teeth to the ideal position as orthodontist plans for patients. Bracket bonding and wire ligation are not needed. So most people may not notice you are receiving orthodontic treatment.

However, with this kind of aligners, it is almost impossible to move teeth precisely. This appliance is not applicable for all patients. It may be useful for only simple tooth movement. Because this appliance looks very simple and invisible, many patients come to ask about it. Visiting dental clinic for asking this appliance seems to be very helpful for increasing the number of orthodontic patients.

32. Tooth Brushing Instruction

A. Importance of Brushing the Teeth

B. Tooth Brushing Instruction Using Disclosing Solution

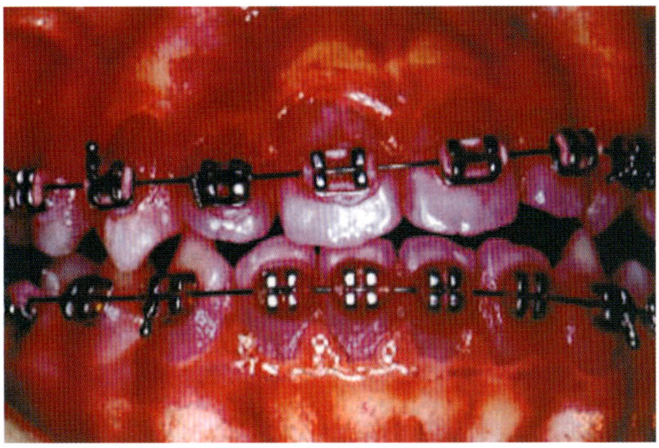

A. Importance of Brushing the Teeth

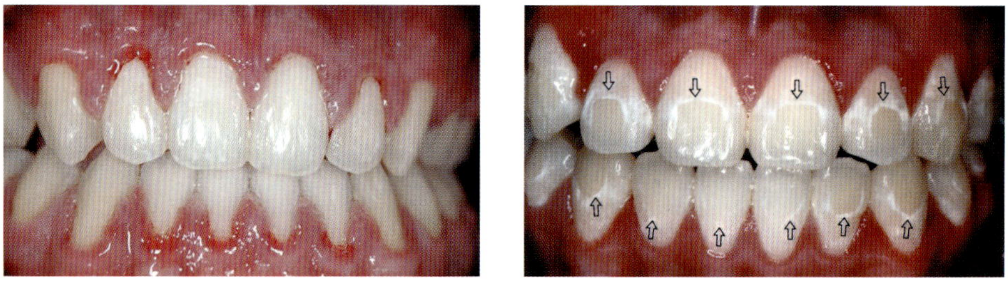

Neglecting tooth brushing during treatment resulted in gum disease(left) and decayed teeth(arrows on right photo)

If brushing the teeth is neglected during the treatment period, the teeth will become decayed or resulted in gum diseases at the end of treatment, making the treatment completely useless. If the child is not at an age when she/he can brush the teeth perfectly for oneself, then it is best to postpone the treatment.

B. Tooth Brushing Instruction Using Disclosing Solution

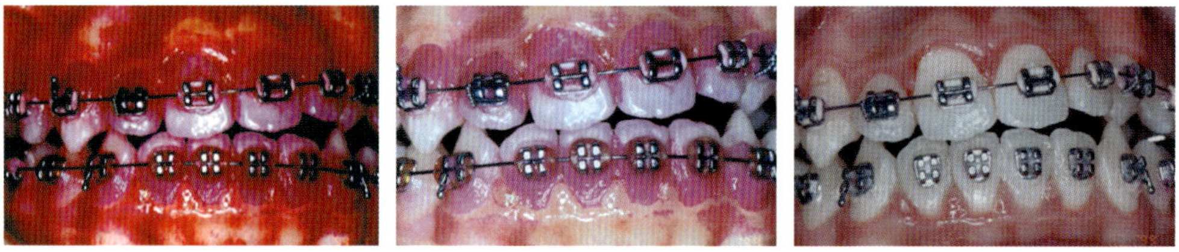

before brushing incomplete brushing just after thorough brushing

After placing the brackets, the brushing technique is explained to the patient. After having the patient gargle with red liquid dye called "disclosing solution", a mirror is used to show where the dye is most largely left.

It is easy for food particles to get trapped in the bracket. Liquid dye is used to show where the food particles get trapped the most. Brushing the teeth after placement of brackets is much different from normal brushing.

Therefore, even the children who were good at brushing their teeth should use the liquid dye to show where the brushing had been missed. Whether brushing the teeth completely or not depends not on age but on personality, so it must get used to be a good habit of brushing after meal from an early age.

IX. Pain Associated with Orthodontic Treatment

33. Pain during Tooth Movement

A. Histological Structure of Alveolar Bone

B. How Can Hard Tooth Move?

C. Process of Tooth Movement

D. Adequate Force for Tooth Movement

E. Pain Associated with Orthodontic Treatment

F. Is it Possible to Receive Treatment without Pain?

G. There Are Appliances that Are Completely Painless.

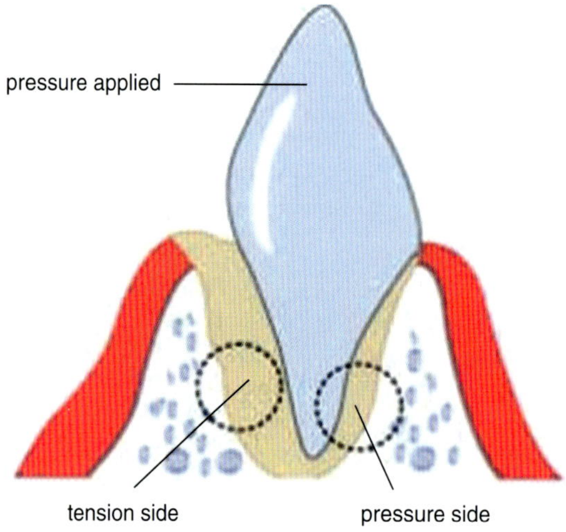

A. Histological Structure of Alveolar Bone

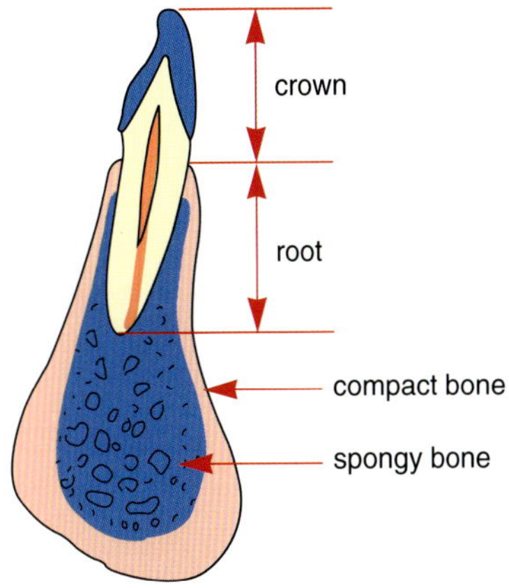

Alveolar(tooth) bone around the root of tooth is made up of spongy bone.

Histologically, the tooth is made up of cancellous bones, which are much like sponges. If you push down the tooth, it will sink, but when you let it go, it will return to its original position. Of course, it's so small amounts that it cannot be noticed by the naked eye, or tactile senses.

B. How Can Hard Teeth Move?

There are some people say that "I don't believe that teeth can move", because they think bones are as hard as rock, and teeth are as hard as porcelain. With this in mind, it is understandable why some peoples have doubts about it.

Although the bone is hard, it has blood supply within it, and it is composed of cells just like other tissues in the body. Thus, it carries on biological activities such as cell division, development, growth, and proliferation.

Cells are considered as the smallest unit of life. Since human body is composed of living cells, the bone is also considered as alive. So it is quite natural for the teeth to move in response to the force generated from the appliance.

C. Process of Tooth Movement

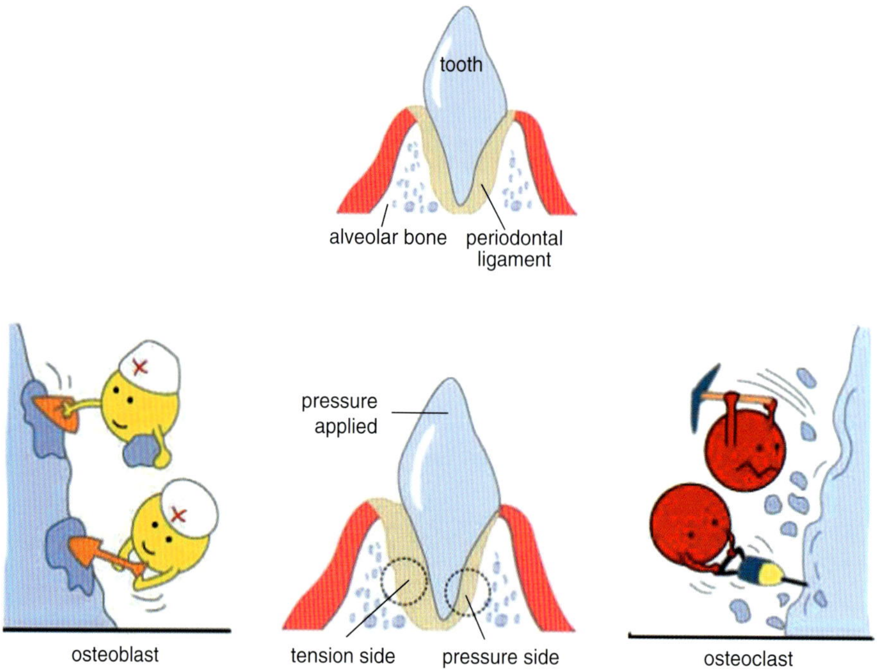

Tooth imbedded in alveolar(tooth socket) bone. If pressure applies to the tooth, tension and pressure zone appears. Osteoblast on the tension zone forms new bone, and osteoclast on the pressure zone resorbs alveolar bone.

When force is applied to the tooth, cells in both the periodontal ligament and alveolar(tooth socket) bone will proliferate. The periodontal ligament receiving the pressure will make cells called osteoclasts. Their function is to resorb the bone, then on the other zone that is receiving the traction, cells called osteoblasts appear and they will form bones. As a result, after four to five hours, the tooth will start to move.

If the force applied to the tooth is too weak, it will not move and if it is too strong, it will resorb the root or on the contrary, retard the moving activity.

D. Adequate Force for Tooth Movement

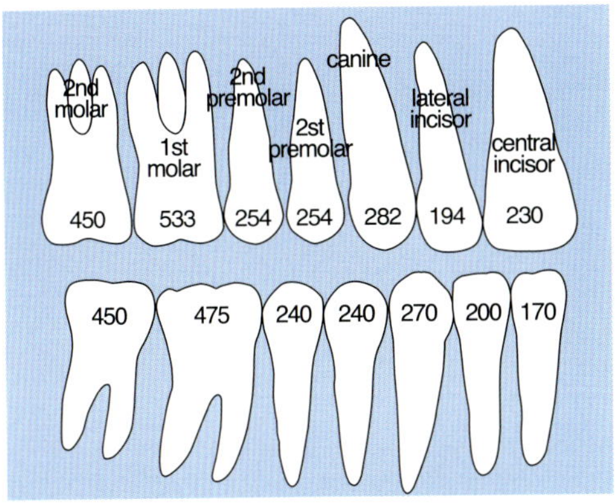

This drawing shows the amount of force needed for each tooth movement. If the tooth is big enough to have a greater root surface area, then more force is needed(Modified from Proffit WR. Contemporary Orthodontics 2nd ed. St. Louis, 1993 Mosby-Yearbook).

In order for the tooth to move properly, the cell's activity must be adequate and for this, the force applied to each tooth must be decided in proportion to the surface area of the root.

The smallest tooth, which is the lower front teeth needs approximately 170g, and the teeth with the longest single root, the canine, needs 282g.

E. Pain Associated with the Orthodontic Treatment

If pressure is applied to a tooth, pain develops as the periodontal ligament is compressed. For almost all patients, the pain associated with the initial activation of the appliance is the most severe.

There is a great deal of individual variation for pain experience. Some patients report little or no pain, whereas others experience considerable pain under the same conditions. The pain generally lasts for 2 to 4 days, then disappears until the orthodontic appliance is reactivated after a month.

After monthly reactivation, patient may feel pain several hours later, but pain usually disappears soon. The patient feels only mild discomforts after monthly reactivation.

F. Is it possible to receive treatment without pain?

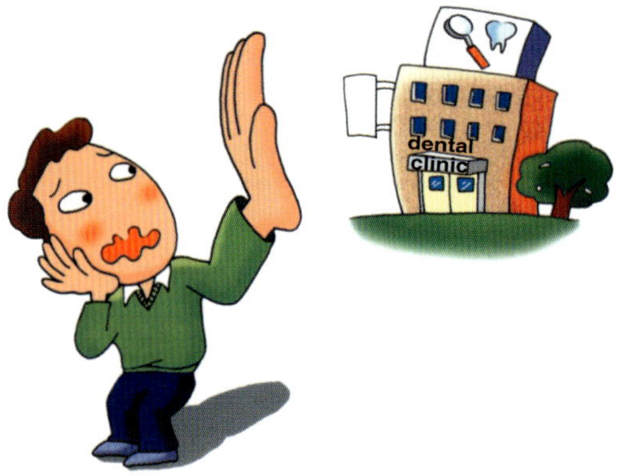

Pain in itself is a biological defense mechanism for all the animal. Some people postpone the orthodontic treatment because of fear of pain. Normally, if you are careful enough to eat soft foods for 2 to 3 days after placement of the orthodontic appliance, the pain should be minimized and uncomfortable feelings of wearing the appliances should also disappear completely within a week.

During the orthodontic treatment, a monthly visit to the orthodontist is required. At this time the orthodontic appliances are adjusted and changed, and then some people may feel pain for 2 to 3 days.

However, the pain patients feel at this time is much less than the pain felt at the beginning, so there is no need to refrain from enjoying various type of foods. You feel relieved if you think the teeth are moving within the bone. Slight pain or discomfort is inevitable when moving the teeth.

G. There are appliances that are completely painless.

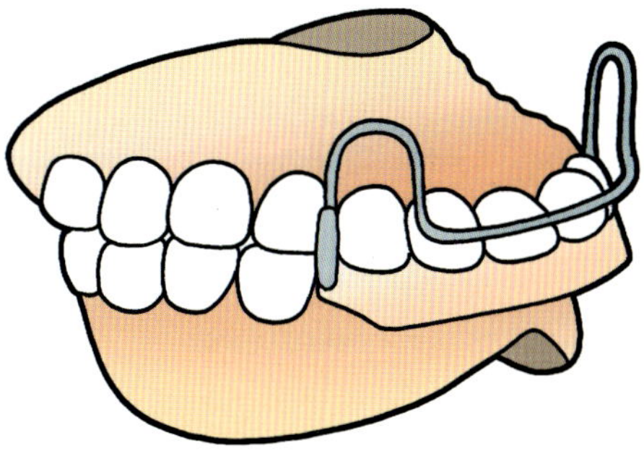

Among the orthodontic appliances, there are some appliances that do not use the artificial force generated from orthodontic appliance such as wire, coil spring, or elastics. Instead, they utilize the force from muscles in the mouth. They are called "functional orthopedic appliance". This appliance uses natural force to control the growth and development of jaw bones or move the teeth; therefore, there is no pain or discomfort.

However, since this appliance utilizes the natural forces generated from the soft tissues, it is not possible to move each tooth precisely. Therefore, this kind of appliance is not applicable for all patients.

This type of appliances are mainly used for growth modification during the growth and development period. It is also used as retainers after orthodontic treatment.

X. Orthodontic Treatment in Reality

34. Examination and Diagnosis Materials

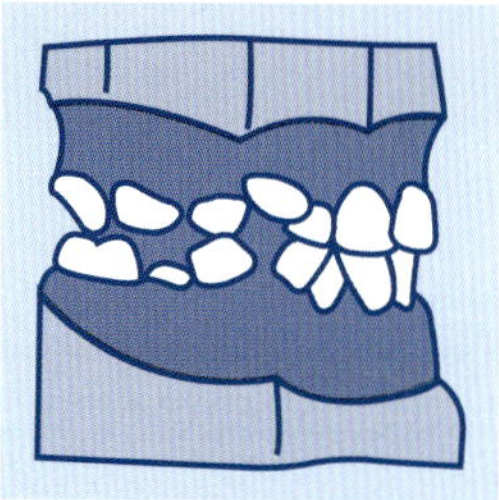

1. Study Model

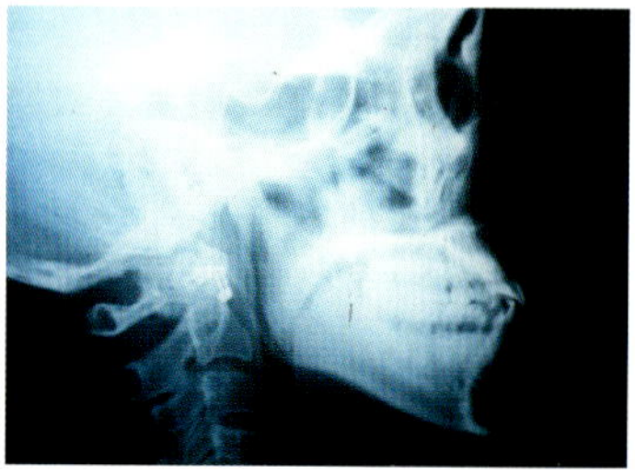

2. Cephalography

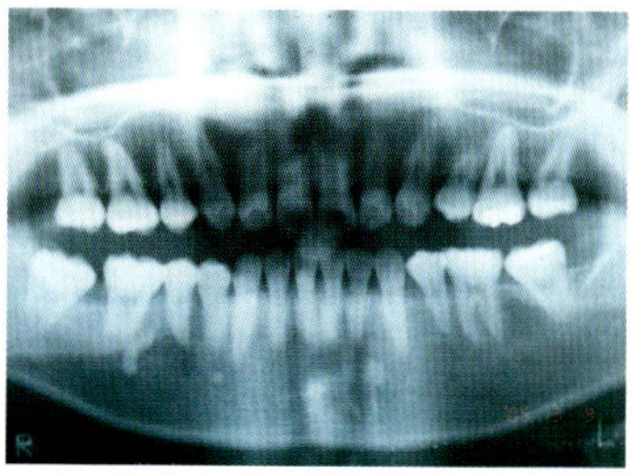

3. Panorama

1. Study Model

With the upper and lower teeth are set together, the position and the size of the teeth, and the width and length of the upper and lower dentitions are examined accurately.

2. Cephalography

Position of the lower and upper jaw, the relationship between the teeth and the jaws, and prediction of the growth and development of the upper and lower jaws are examined.

3. Panorama

The condition of the teeth contained in the alveolar bone is examined to determine the existence of congenital missing teeth, and the abnormality in the both jaws. Abnormal temporomandibular(jaw) joint is also examined.

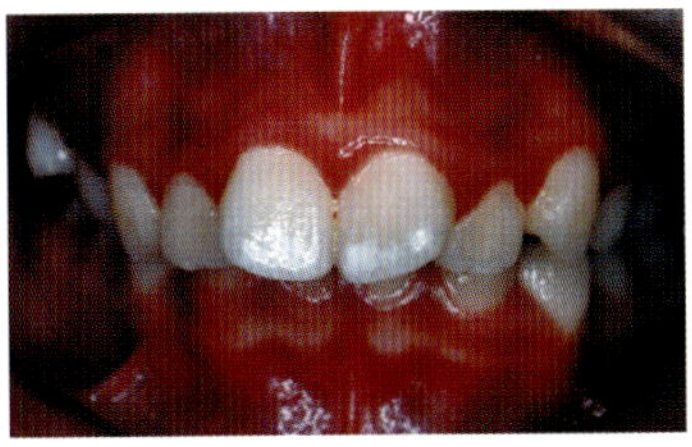

4. Intraoral photos.

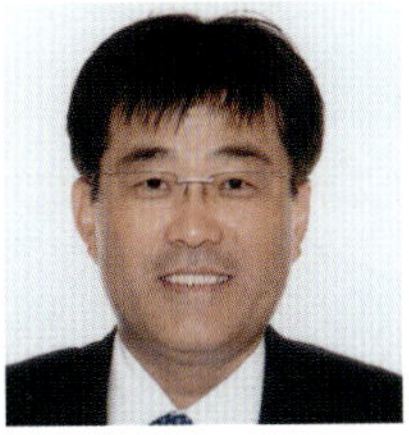

5. Facial Photos.

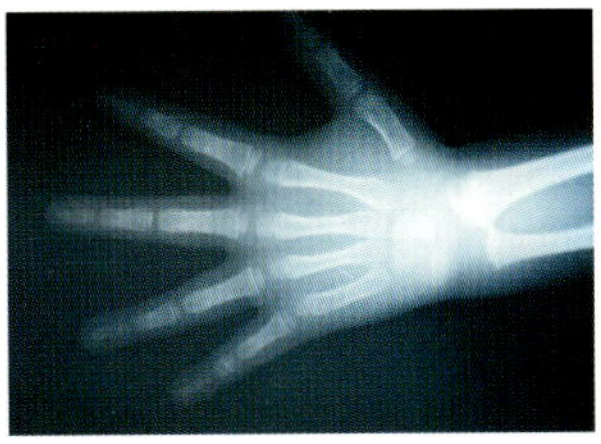

6. Hand & Wrist Photos

4. Intraoral photos

Examine the conditions of each tooth, gums, and compare between before and after treatment status.

5. Facial Photos

Examine the shape of the lips, the overall proportion, and the changes in the profile that take place during the treatment.

6. Hand & Wrist Photos

It is used to estimate the remaining growth and development of the face in a patient who is still growing.

35. Procedures for Orthodontic Treatment

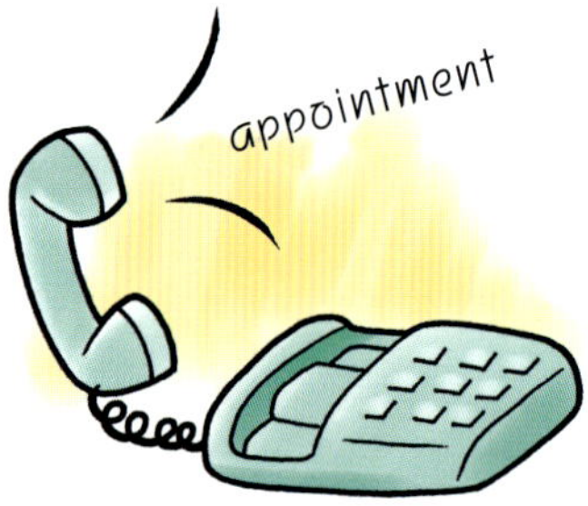

1. Appointment

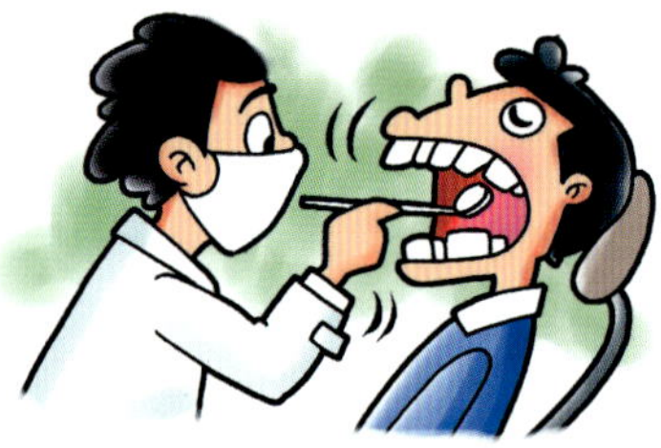

2. Visit and Examination

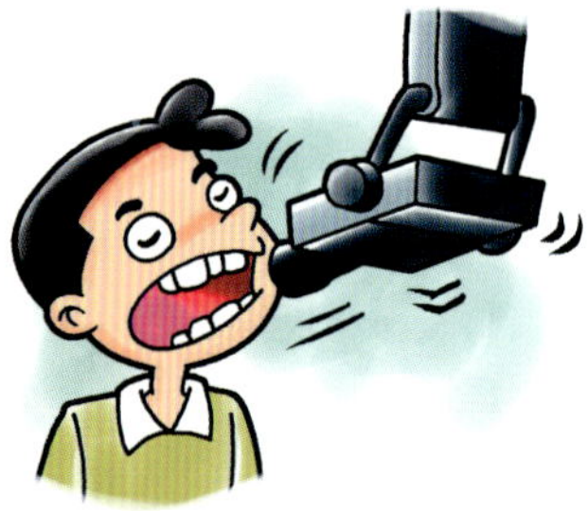

3. X-ray, Study Model, Photo

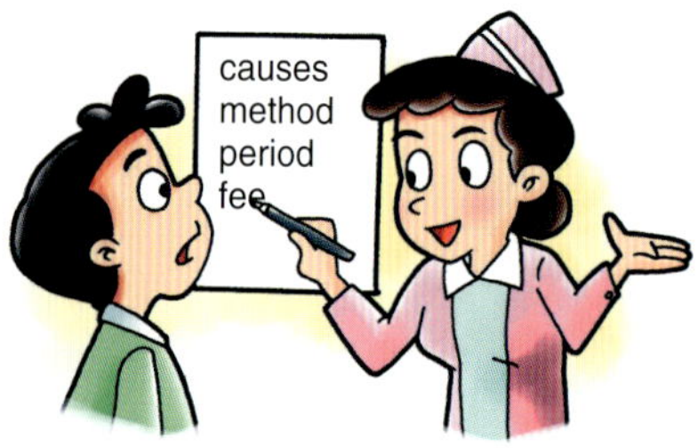

4. Explanation of Treatment

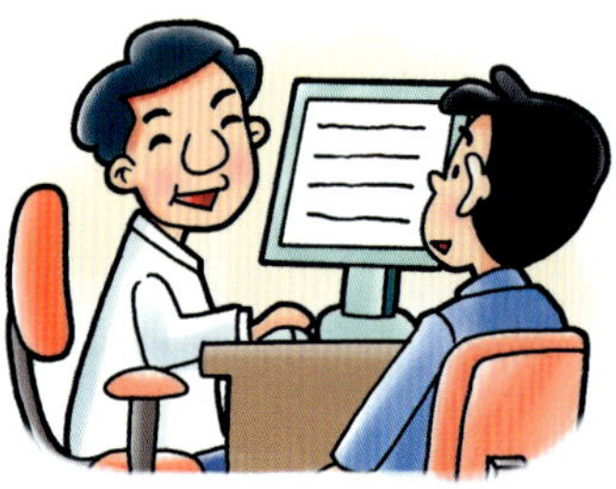

5. Explanation of Treatment Schedule

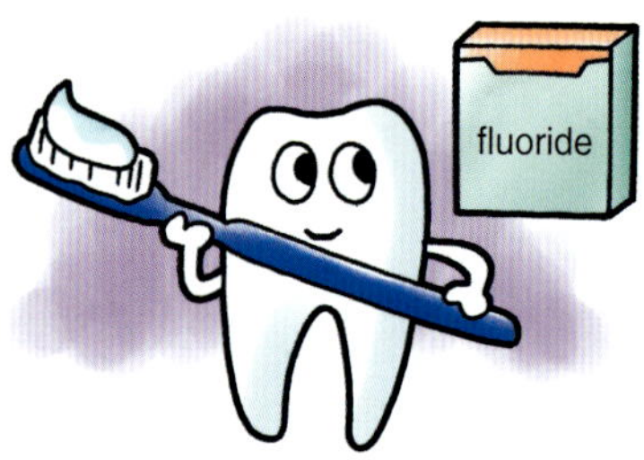

6. Preventive Treatment for Caries Control

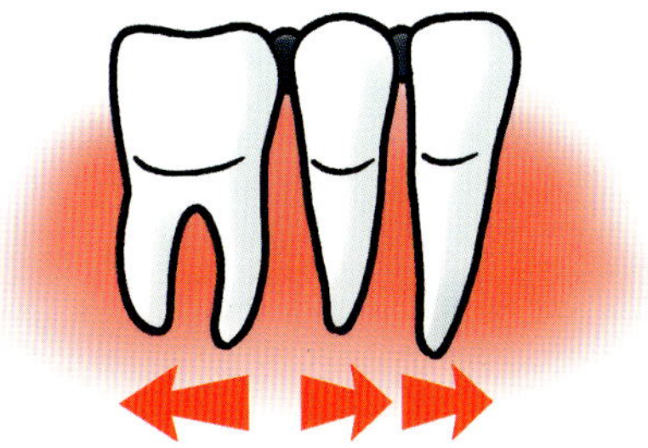

7. Rubber Ring Placement for Band Space

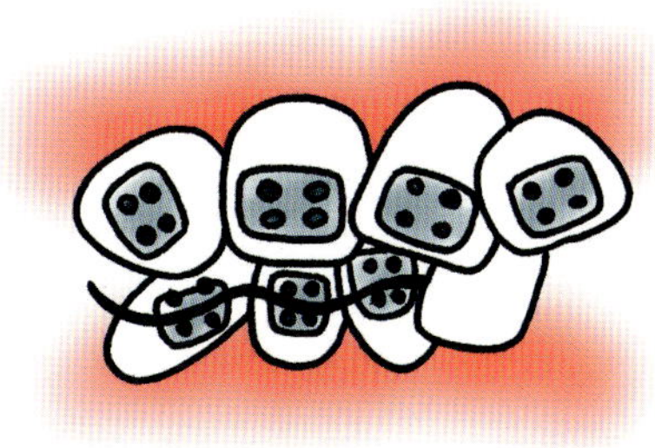

8. Bracket Bonding

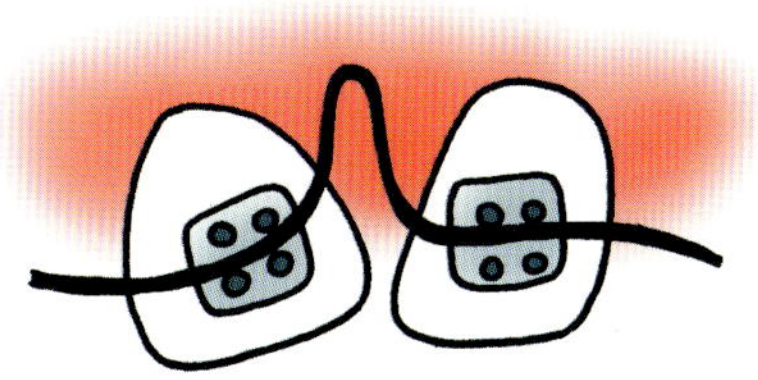

9. Placement of Orthodontic Wire

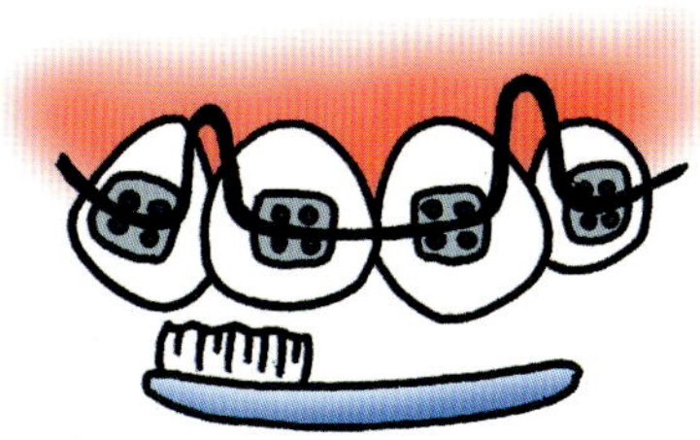

10. Tooth Brushing Instruction

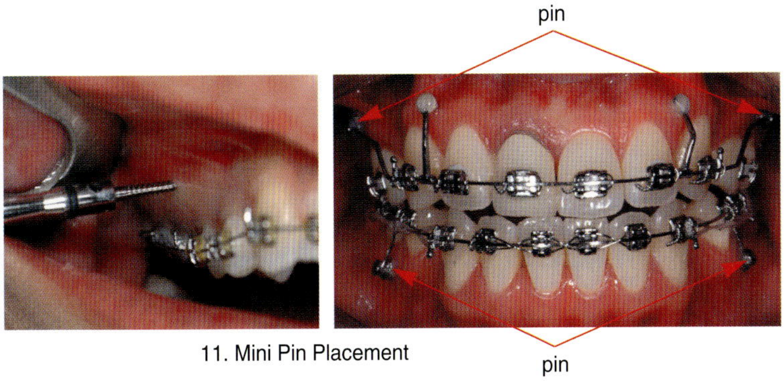

11. Mini Pin Placement

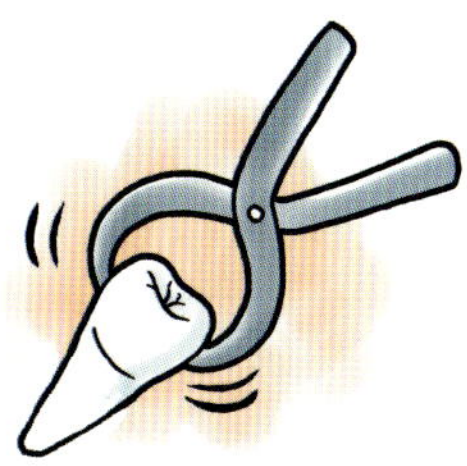

12. Removal of Teeth if Necessary

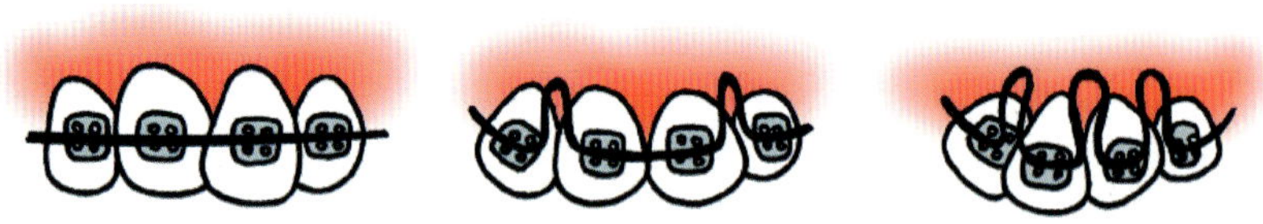

13. Monthly Visiting for Appliance Adjustment

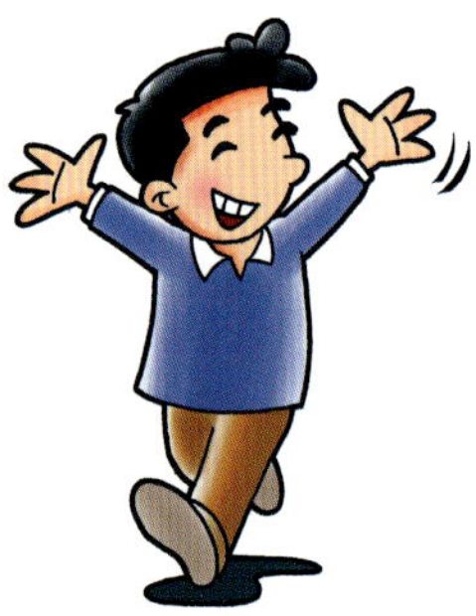

14. Finished Active Treatment

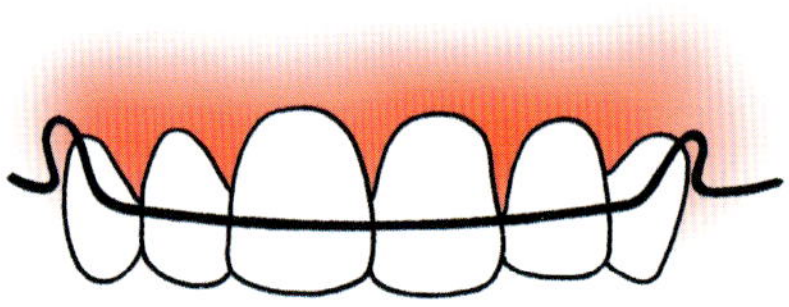

15. After the brackets are removed, removable retainers are worn to maintain the new position of the teeth.

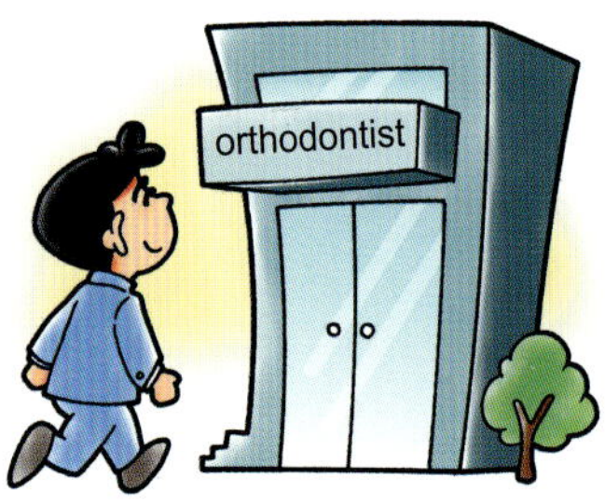

16. Periodic Check-up

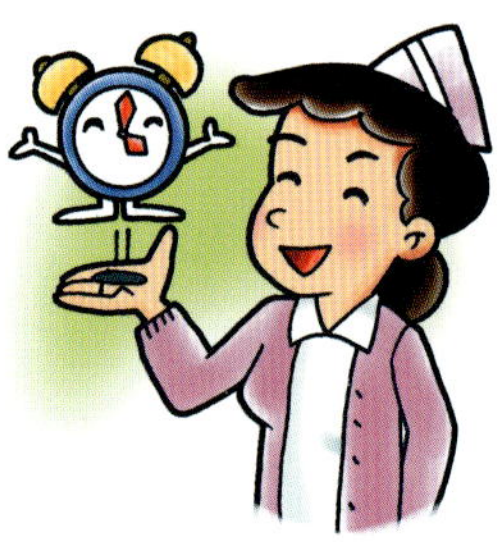

17. The duration of the treatment differs according to the patient's condition.

36. Matters that Demand Special Attention during Treatment

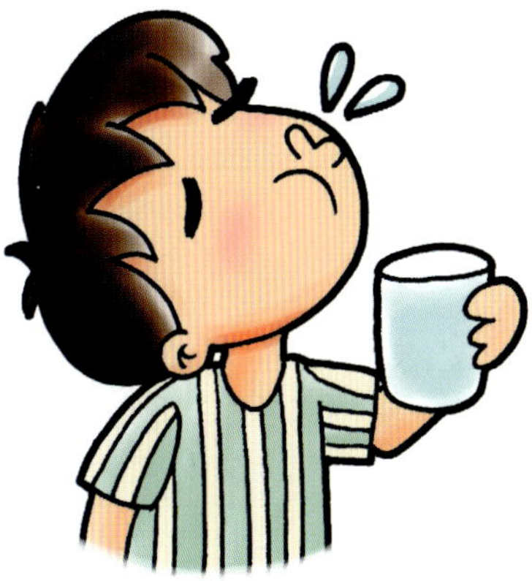

1. Slight pain can be appeared after first placement of orthodontic appliance or monthly adjustment of orthodontic arch wire. It disappears little by little with lapse of time. Gargling with a cup of luke warm water contained a spoonful salt will relieve this pain.

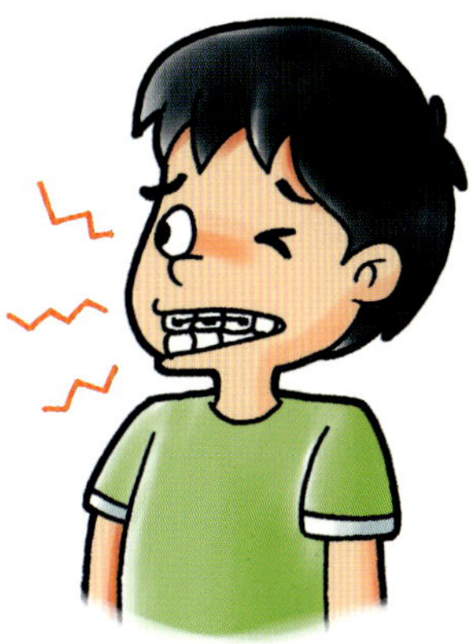

2. At first time you wear orthodontic appliance, you have difficulties in speaking, eating, and swallowing, but it disappears within 2 or 3 days.

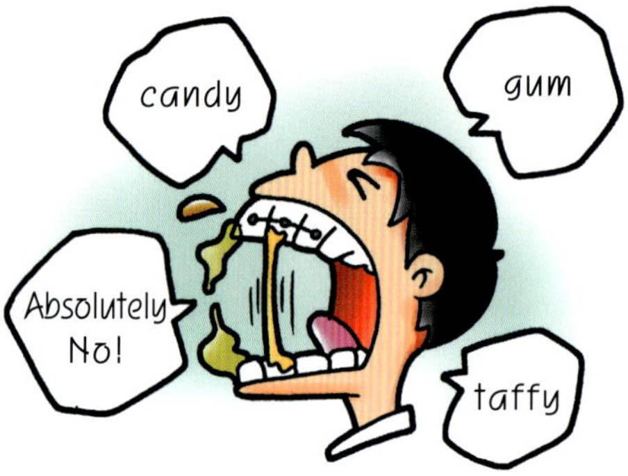
candy
gum
Absolutely No!
taffy

3. Don't take sticky food materials such as chewing gum, caramel, wheat gluten. If you take these kinds of food, orthodontic appliance will get broken or deformed.

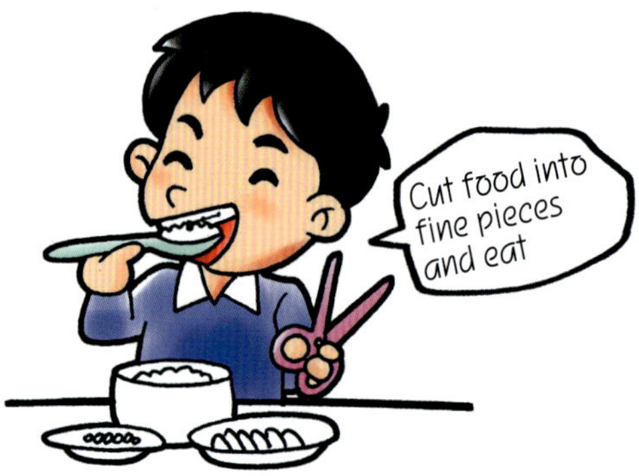
Cut food into fine pieces and eat

4. If you eat tough foods such as meat, Kimchi, and large-sized food materials such as apple, pear, and hamburger etc, you must cut them into fine pieces.

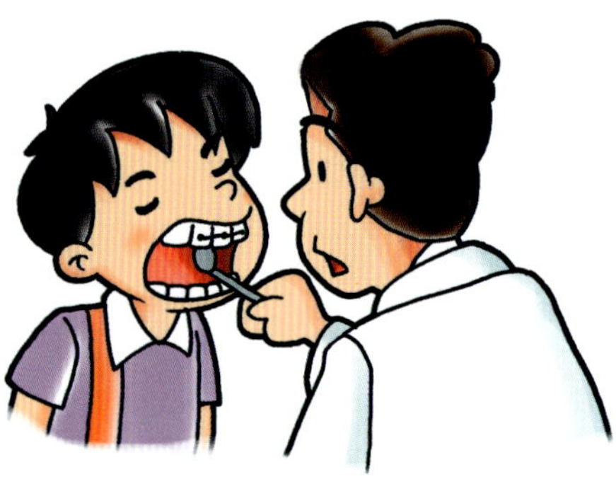

5. If severe pains continue, band is loosened, bracket is detached, orthodontic elastics can't be worn, and/or forget the position where the elastics are hung, you must visit orthodontist as soon as possible.

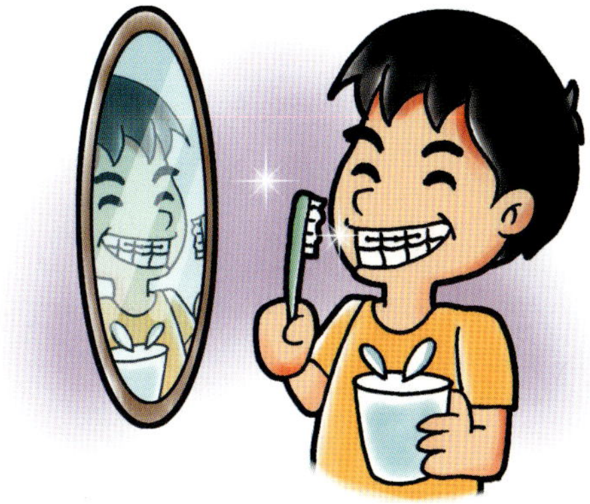

6. When the orthodontic appliances such as brackets, wires, tubes, coil springs etc are placed on the teeth, food particles are easily trapped. Therefore, you must brush your teeth thoroughly after each meal. Check the brushing using mirror. If you neglect brushing the teeth during orthodontic treatment, you will have decayed teeth, bleeding gums, and bad mouth breath.

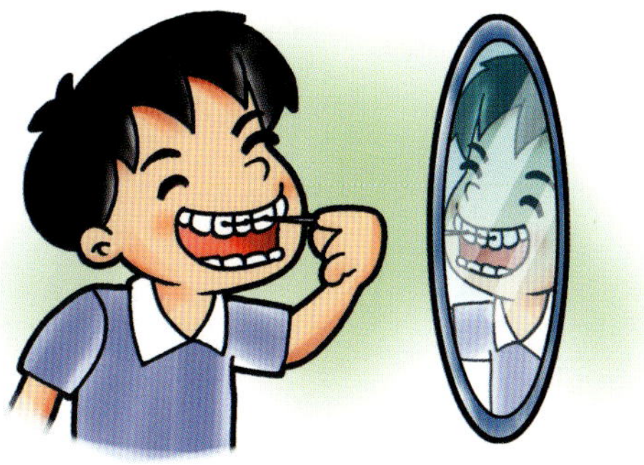

7. If you have difficulties in removing food particles packed in orthodontic appliance, you can use tooth pick or small-sized brush named proxabrush given from a dental clinic. Be careful not to hurt gum or not to get broken the appliance.

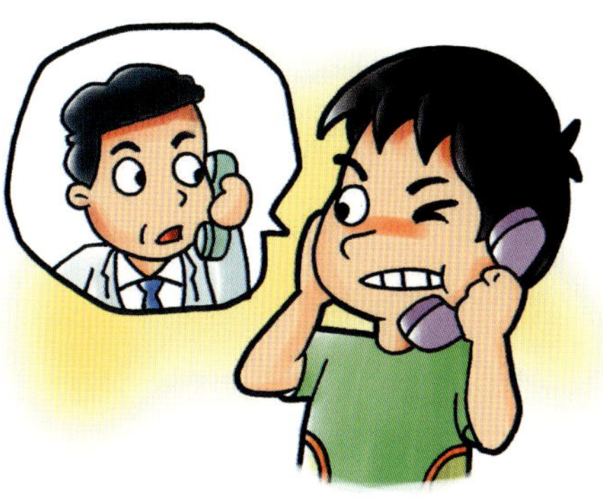

8. If orthodontic wire is pierced into soft tissue and pain appeared, cover that region with cotton, and then visit a doctor as soon as possible.

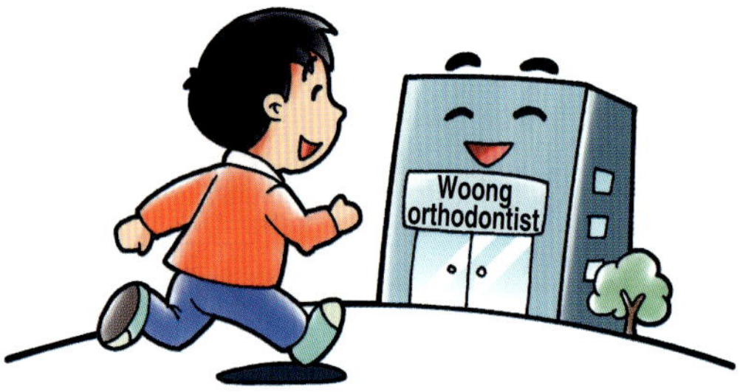

9. Keep the appointment day.

XI. Prevention of Malocclusions

37. To Prevent Bad Alignment of Teeth

A. Consult Your Dentist Beforehand

B. Regular Check-Ups

C. Early Sign of Bad Alignment of Teeth

D. Stop Bad Habits as soon as Possible

E. Treat the Cavities as soon as Possible

F. Results of Early Loss of Milk Tooth

G. Space Maintainer

H. Primate Space

I. Sparsely Aligned Children's Front Teeth

J. No Developmental Space

K. Over-retained Milk Teeth

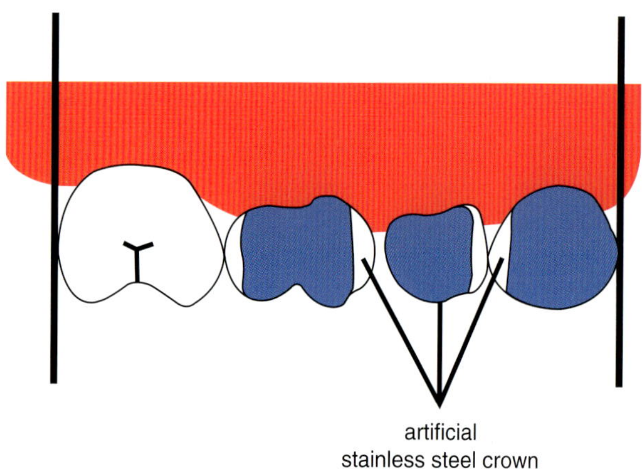

A. Consult Your Family Dentist Beforehand

Although there seems to be no problems with the teeth alignment, it is recommended that you receive consultation for orthodontic problems regularly. This is possibly to prevent the teeth alignment from getting worse.

As your children receive regular physical check-ups, if they are at an age when they should be thinking about proper teeth alignment, it is a good idea to get a consult from a family dentist.

This way, it will be possible to manage their teeth so that it does not erupt badly. If, however, they have already badly erupted, then the appropriate treatment can be started.

B. Regular Check-ups

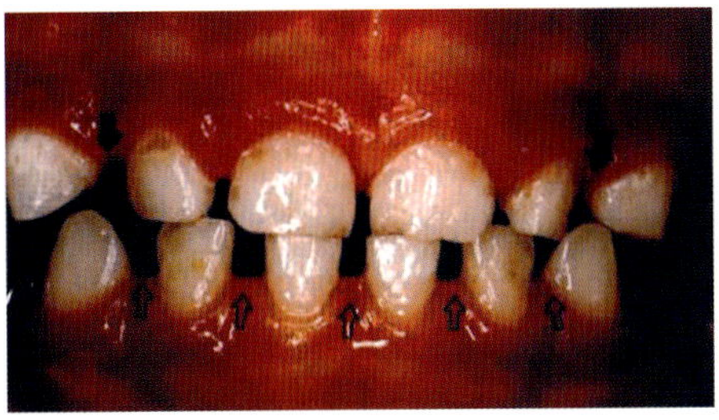

It is normal for a children's teeth to erupt sparsely. When the permanent teeth erupt, the space will disappear and good alignment of adult teeth will be attained.

C. Early Sign of Bad Alignment of Teeth

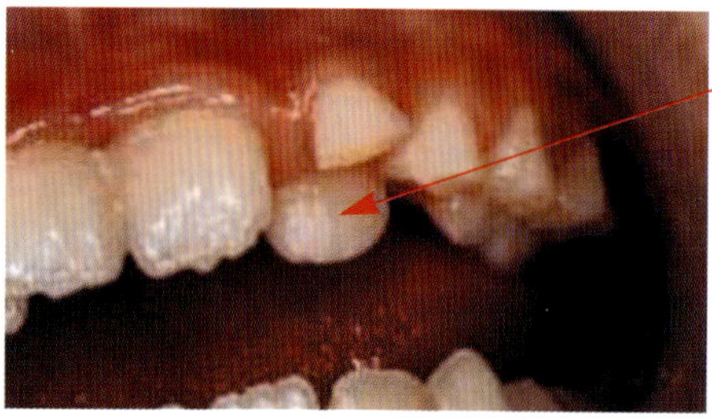

abnormally erupted lateral incisor

Since there are no spaces between the milk teeth, the permanent teeth are erupted sideways. There is a higher possibility for the teeth to become crooked.

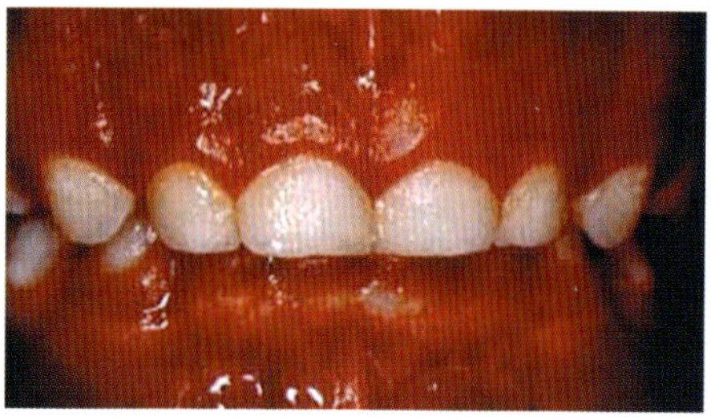

Also, since the upper incisors(front teeth) are covering the lower incisors completely, it is likely for the upper teeth to be protruded. Therefore, regular check-up is necessary at an early ages.

D. Stop Bad Habits as soon as Possible

Also bad alignment of teeth may develop from bad habits such as sucking the thumb or biting the finger nails, so it is best to have these habits stopped before the age of 4 or 5.

E. Treat Cavities as soon as Possible

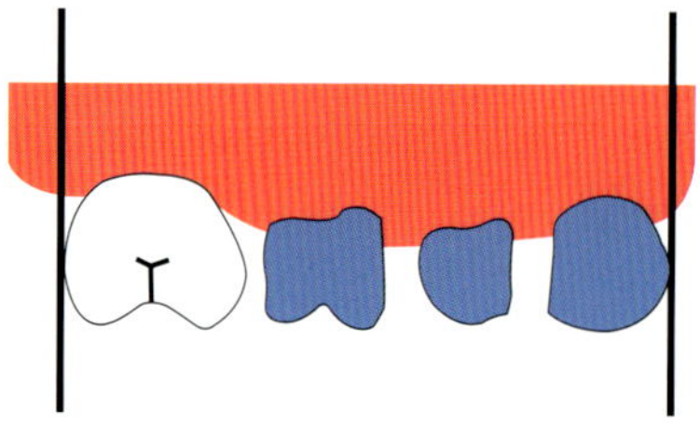

The width of the tooth has already decreased because of cavities.

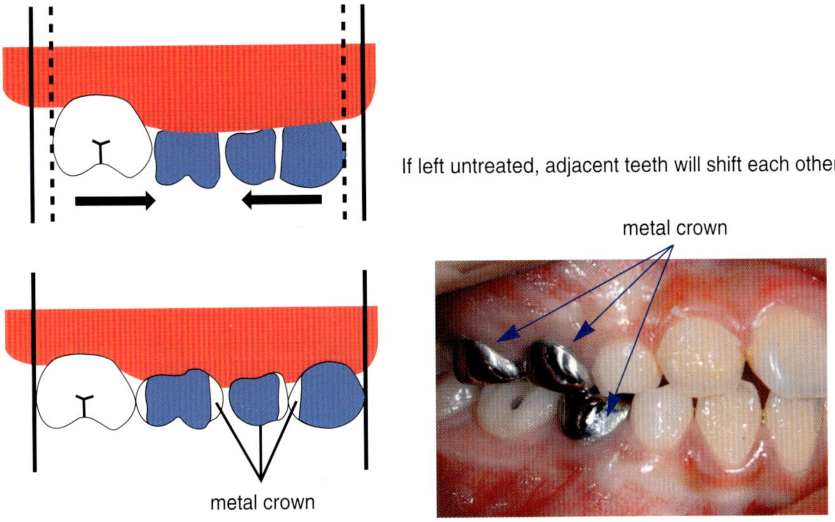

To prevent the shifting of the teeth, cavities must be treated immediately to keep the original width. Arrows mean metal crown.

Although we cannot prevent the size differences between the upper and lower jaw or, the oversize and the undersize of the teeth in comparison with the alveolar(tooth) bone, there are some cases where prevention is possible.

Cavities can cause the tooth to change the direction of its eruption or bad alignment of teeth may develop because of the loss of eruption space. Therefore, you must be careful not to develop cavities. If cavities already occurred, cavities must be restored to the original tooth width.

F. Result of Early Loss of Milk Tooth

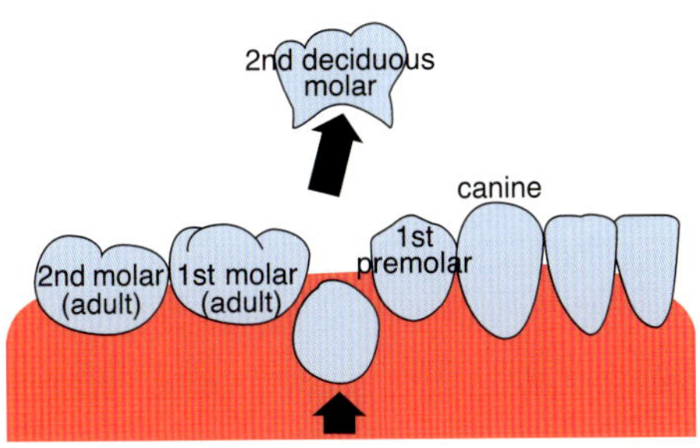

If the adult back tooth(first molars) has shifted forward because of severe cavities of deciduous molars(milk back tooth) during the mixed dentition or if there is a lack of space to erupt, then the canine teeth of upper jaw will be crooked or second premolar of the lower jaw may not be able to erupt.

Therefore, in case of premature loss of milk back tooth, consultation with an orthodontist is necessary.

G. Space Maintainer

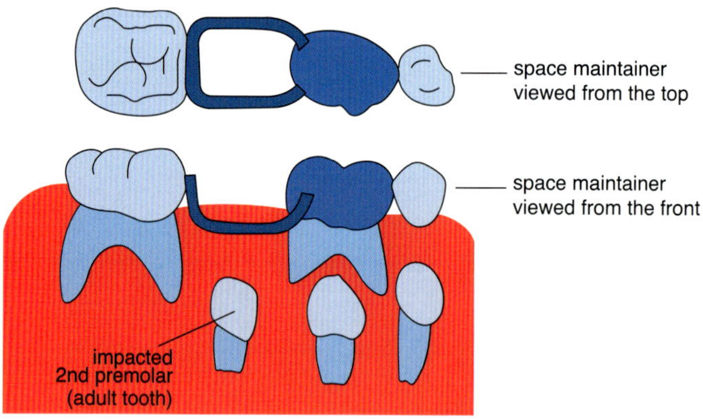

If the second deciduous molar(milk back tooth) is removed earlier than usual because of caries, then the first molar which is already erupted will shift forward and the permanent second premolar will not be able to erupt.

If the deciduous molar is missed too early, then a space maintainer must be inserted to secure space for the permanent premolar which is still being developed in the alveolar bone.

H. Primate Space

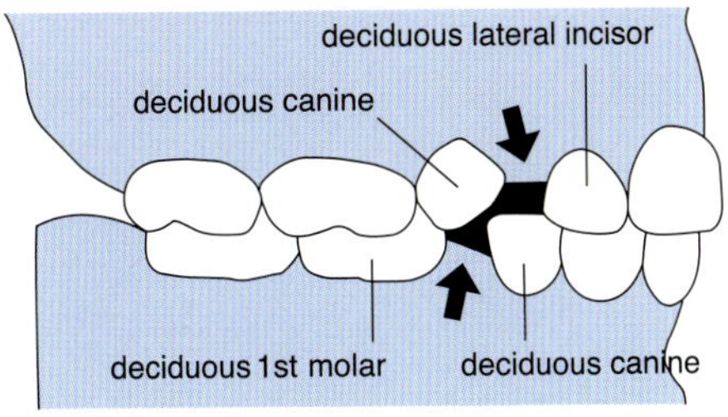

human

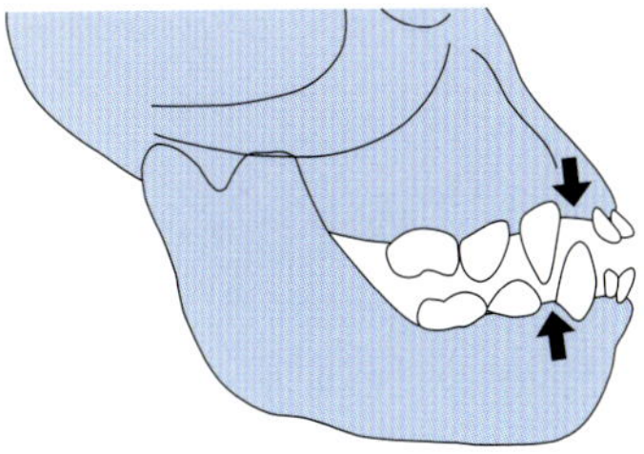

ape

It is normal for the primary dentition to align sparsely. Especially noticeable spaces are existed in two locations of a primary dentition. In the upper jaw, space exists between the deciduous lateral incisors and the canines. Whereas, in the lower jaw, there are some spaces between the deciduous canines and the first molars.

These two spaces are called primate space. As the name indicates, in most sub-human primates such as apes have these characteristic spaces throughout life. Normally, the primate space will disappear at the time of the eruption of the permanent adult teeth.

I. Sparsely Aligned Children's Front Teeth

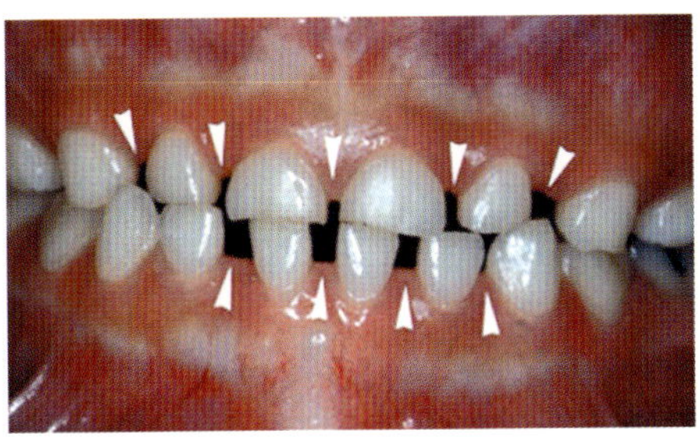

The space between the children's front teeth is called the developmental spaces. Developmental spaces are often present from when the teeth start to erupt, but become somewhat larger as the alveolar bone becomes bigger with growth and disappear with the eruption of the permanent adult teeth.

The developmental space in primary dentition is necessary for an ideal alignment of the permanent dentition. Statistically 70% appears in the upper teeth and 63% in the lower teeth.

J. No Developmental Space

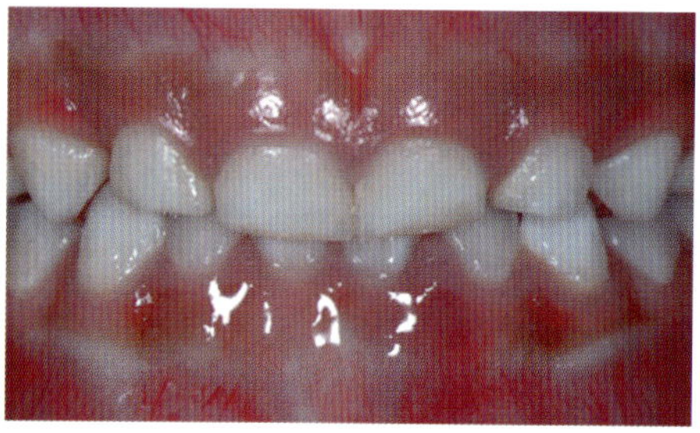

If the children's teeth are good alignment as in this photo, it may look fine, but when the child becomes an adult, there is a high possibility that the teeth will erupt clustered together.

K. Over- retained Milk Teeth

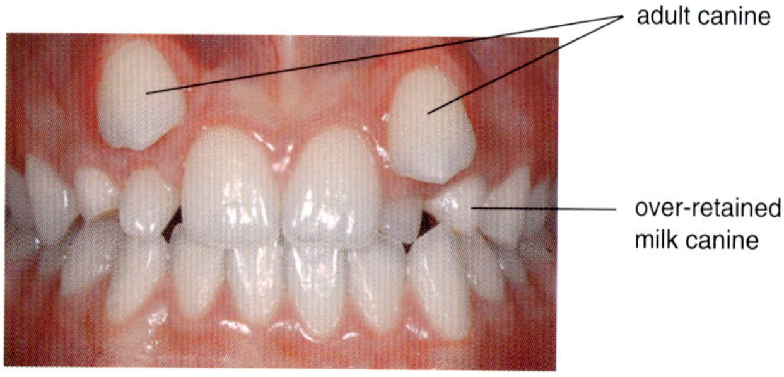

Adult canines are erupted out of position because of prolonged retaining of milk canines. Milk canines should have removed to allow proper positioning of adult canines.

XII. Other Informations about Orthodontic Treatment

38. Orthodontic Specialist

A. Doctor's Obligation

B. Judging the Superiority of the Treatment

C. Orthodontist with Professional Knowledge and Technique

D. Dental Specialty System

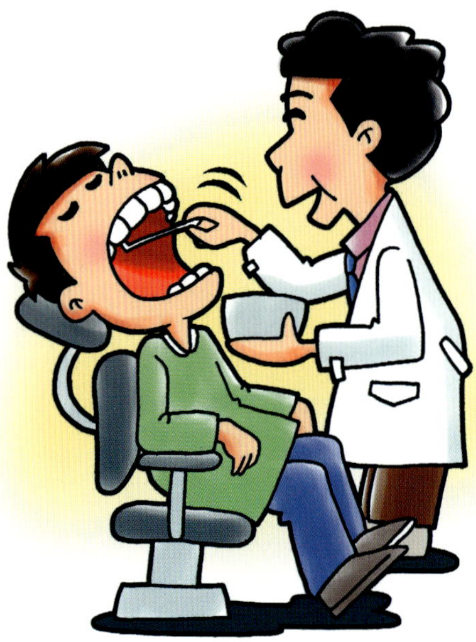

A. Doctor's Obligation

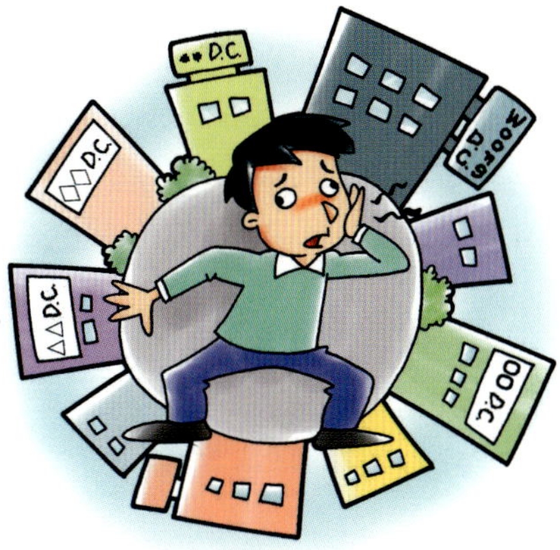

Doctors only have an obligation that equally treat the variety of teeth alignments according to the request of patients with diverse personalities. Since it is the patient's responsibility to choose an orthodontist, some problems can arise.

B. Judging the Superiority of the Treatment

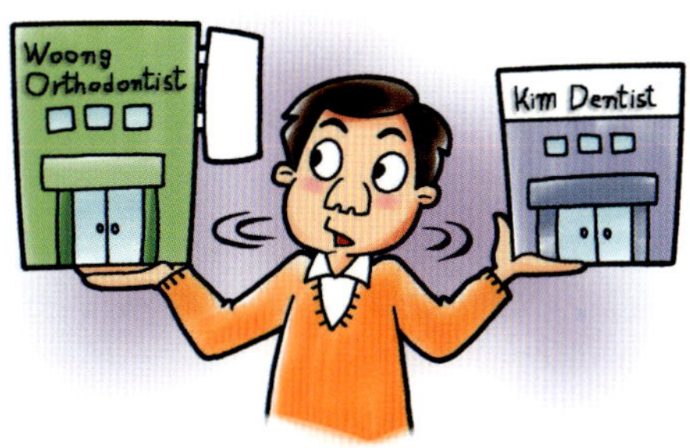

Orthodontics requires advanced knowledge and technology, so it is difficult for the patient to judge the superiority of the treatment skills. Each orthodontist has his own treatment method and philosophy. Therefore, treatment periods, methods for moving tooth, and completion methods etc may vary.

Moving the teeth is one of the conditions required in orthodontic treatment. It only takes up a small portion of the broader orthodontic treatment program. Thus, we should not overlook the patient's condition and overall treatment program by only looking at a small fragment of the treatment.

C. Orthodontist with Professional Knowledge and Technique

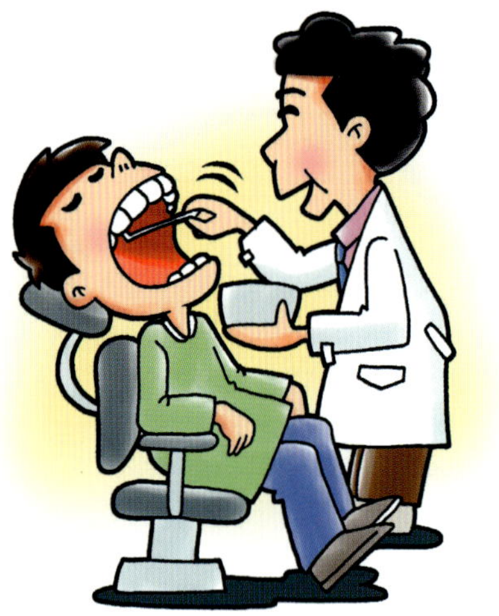

Orthodontic treatment requires professional knowledge, highly specialized technique, and various clinical long experience. Therefore, every dental college and large-scaled private hospital has around 4~5 year's of orthodontic training courses.

Unlike other fields of dentistry, however, orthodontic treatment relatively requires a long term treatment period, which usually starts at adolescence and follows up until adulthood.

This is especially the case since relapse in orthodontics is inevitable whether it is a simple or a severe case. Furthermore, retaining will be required until the end of the growth period or even in some cases for the rest of the patient's life.

Despite these unfavorable conditions, a dentist specializing in orthodontics can be regarded as a person with professional knowledge and confidence in his treatment methods and skills.

D. Dental Specialty System

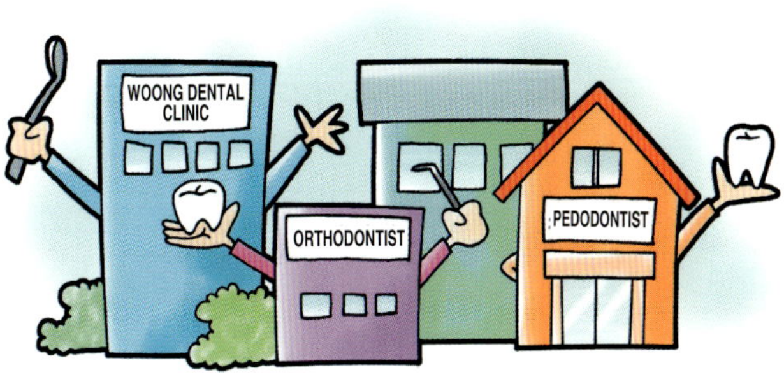

Dental practice system may differ from country to country, but dento-medically advanced countries such as United States, and almost all of wealthy European countries, there are also specialty fields even in dentistry. In order to become a specialist, their professional knowledge must be approved by an official institute.

In Korea, we do not have legislative dental specialty system as in Europe and the United States. Therefore, even orthodontists cannot specify our specialty even though we received several years of orthodontic training.

Therefore, there is much possibilities of choosing a dentist who is not an orthodontic specialist in Korea.

39. Truth about Orthodontic Treatment

A. Do the Teeth That Received Orthodontic Treatment Become Weak?

B. Tooth Must Be Extracted for Orthodontic Treatment.

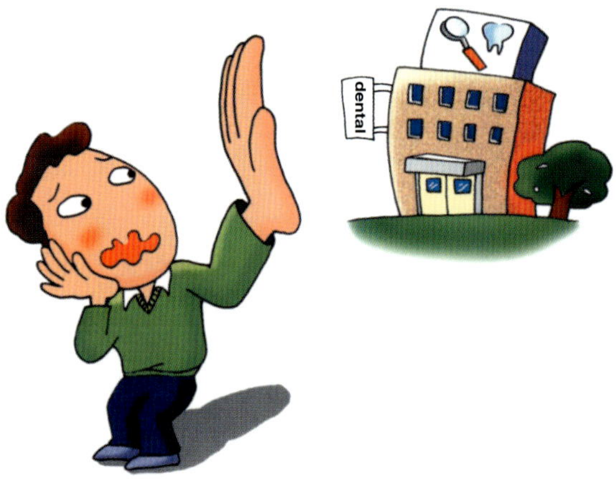

A. Do the Teeth That Received Orthodontic Treatment Become Weak?

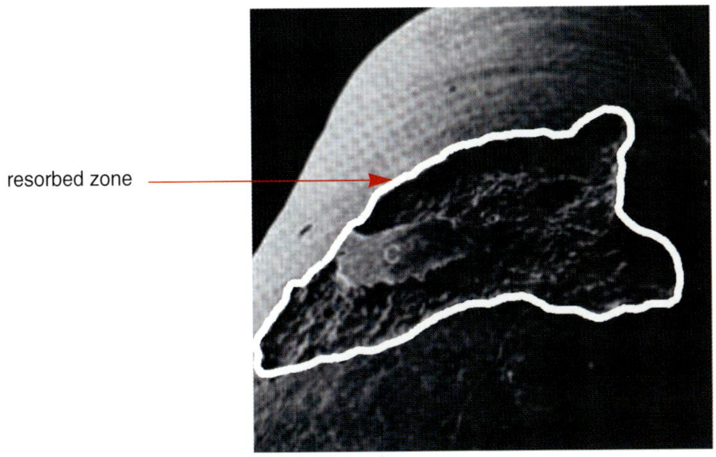

Resorbed root surface after orthodontic treatment
(From Graber, Swain Orthodontics Current Principles and Techniques, 1985, Mosby)

If you take a look at an x-ray picture taken after orthodontic treatment, there may be cases where the end of the root appears to be round because of little bit resorption.

These days, with rapid development in biomedical materials, controlled ideal force can be applied to the tooth during orthodontic treatment, so the resorption of the root has decreased greatly compared to the previous methods.

It is especially important to keep in mind that the metabolism for adults is lower, so the amount of root resorption is greater than children.

After hearing this fact, it is easy to make the mistake of assuming that the teeth will become weak inevitably after treatment, but even without orthodontic treatment, there is normally a slight resorption in the roots.

Even if the root did become resorbed as a result of orthodontic treatment, it would only be a very small amount. Furthermore, it would not have any adverse effects on the external appearance or the function of the teeth.

B. Tooth Must Be Extracted for Orthodontic Treatment.

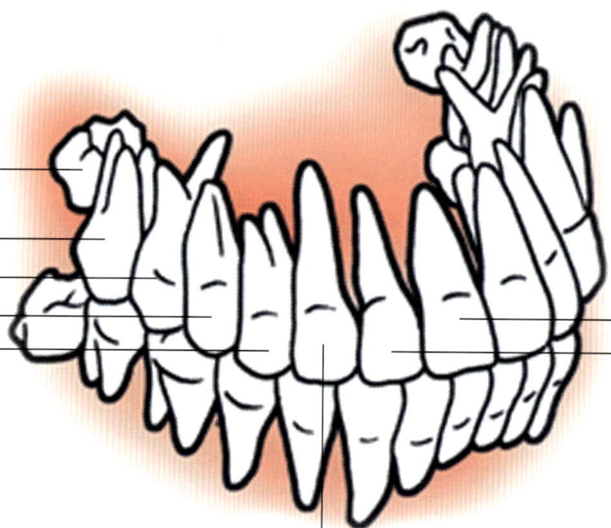

If all 32 teeth are in an ideal alignment, the number of contact points between upper and lower teeth are 132 points, but the premolars only contact in one point. Therefore, these teeth do not play such an important role in chewing. Usually first premolars are extracted.

Also, even if the first premolar is extracted, there is also a 2nd premolar which is almost of the same shape and size will be placed next to the canine after extraction treatment, so it will not be noticeable whether the tooth is missing or not even when you laugh and speak.

Depending on the patient's conditions and form of malocclusion, the 2nd premolar, 2nd molar, or other teeth may be extracted, but whatever the case, the extraction will occur in balance to the right and left side. According to the individual case, there may be cases where only one tooth from the upper jaw or the lower jaw is extracted.

40. Duration of Orthodontic Treatment

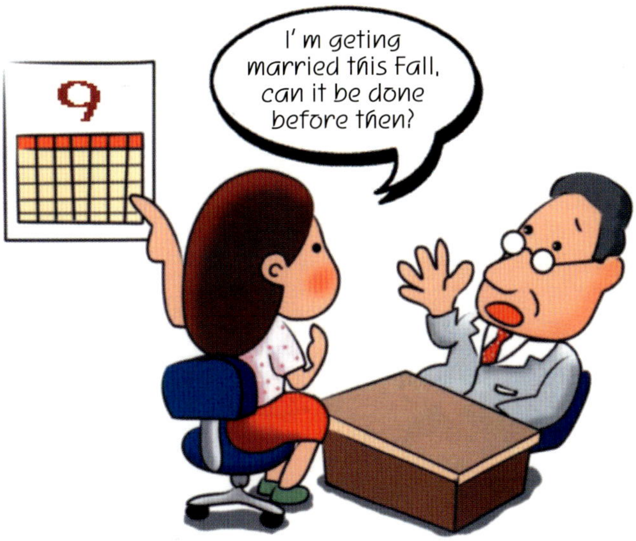

A. In case of the Serial Extraction Technique

Serial Extraction means the selective extraction of deciduous(milk) teeth during the mixed dentition period in accordance with the shedding of the deciduous teeth and eruption of the permanent teeth.

The extraction is accomplished over an extended period of time to ensure the full space for eruption of the lateral incisors, canines, and premolars. Eventually we extract the first premolar teeth for relieving crowding.

For example, if, at an age of 7, the permanent teeth are confirmed to erupt sideways, then the primary teeth can be extracted consecutively prior to the eruption of the permanent teeth to prevent them from erupting sideways. This is called the "Serial Extraction Technique".

Even with this technique, brackets must ultimately be worn for about a year at the age of 12 for precise alignment. Although the treatment period with the brackets is short, the observation period is long, so it can be concluded that the overall treatment period is relatively long.

B. Examples of the Serial Extraction Technique

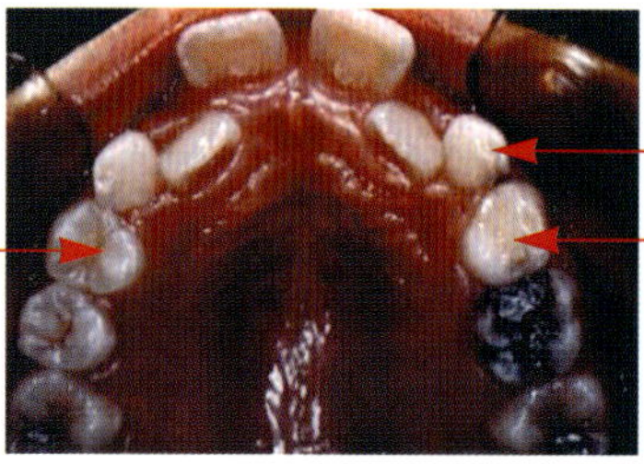

The space for eruption of canine is not sufficient, so it is certain that the canine teeth will erupt sideways. It was decided that the first premolar still in the bone and it should be extracted just after eruption.

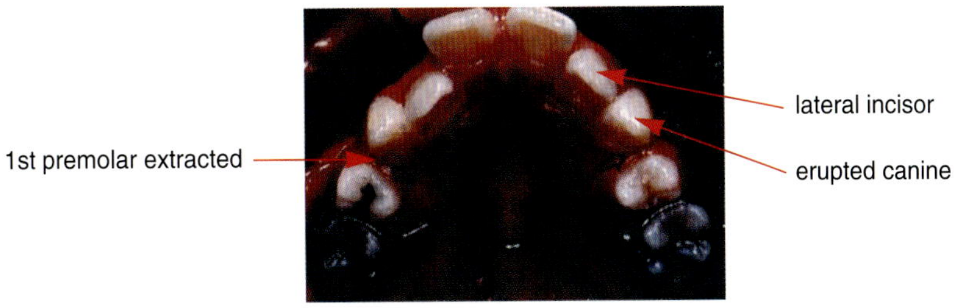

Since the first premolars are extracted beforehand, the rest of the teeth including lateral incisors and canines will have sufficient room for proper alignment.

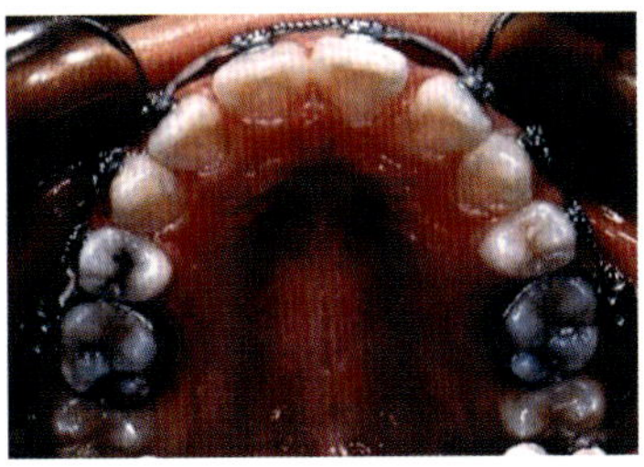

Although the Serial Extraction Technique was used to attain the sufficient room for normal eruption of permanent teeth, the precise teeth alignment does not take place naturally, so brackets are used for one year. The observation and extraction period was longer than the actual orthodontic treatment period.

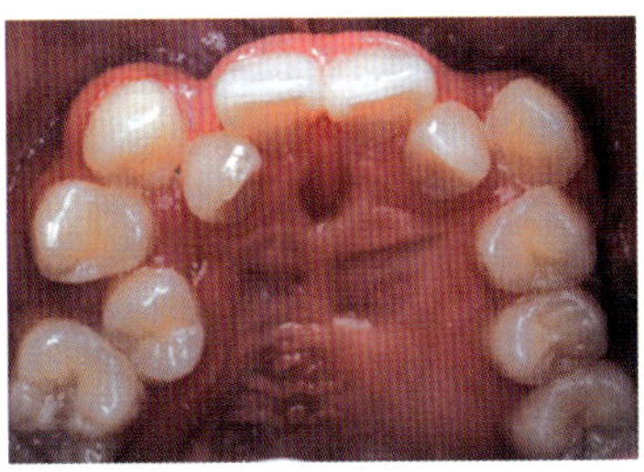

If the Serial Extraction Technique had not been used, the permanent dentition would look like this at the age of 12. It is possible to start treatment with extraction at this time, but since the teeth had already become crooked, there are more chances for a relapse after treatment. Since complete brushing will be difficult, the Serial Extraction Technique is also recommended to prevent permanent teeth from early decaying.

C. Controlling the Growth of the Mandible

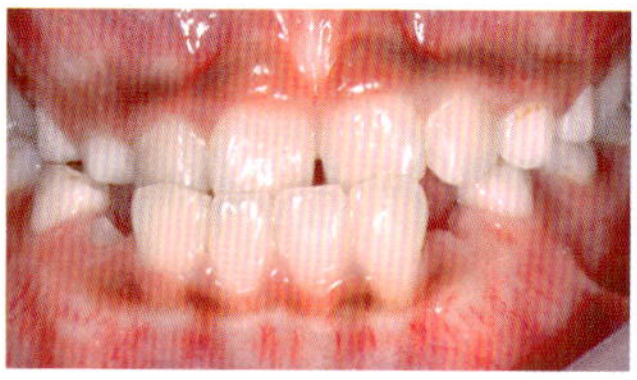
before treatment

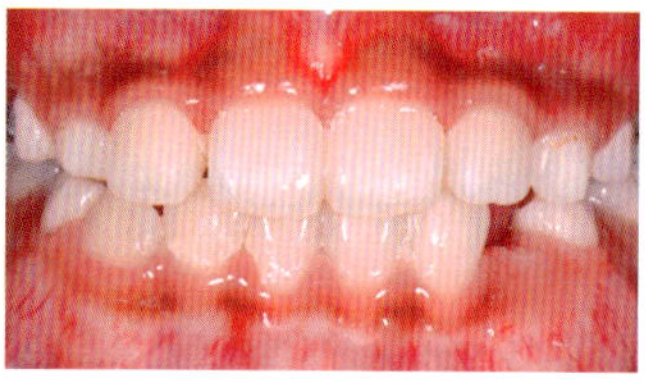
after treatment

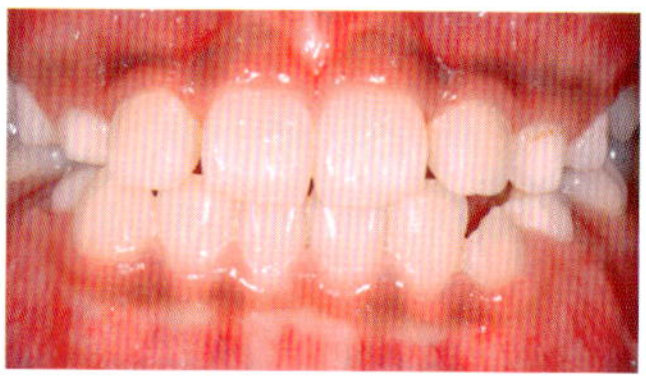
under monitoring

In the case of excessive growth of lower jaw, treatment for inhibiting the growth of the lower jaw at age 5 or 6 can bring ideal results temporarily.

In this case, it is also necessary to observe the patient periodically until the end of the growth period, about ages of 13 for girls and about 18 for boys. If the periodic observation is included in the treatment period, it would take 7 to 8 years.

D. Can the Treatment Period Be Shortened?

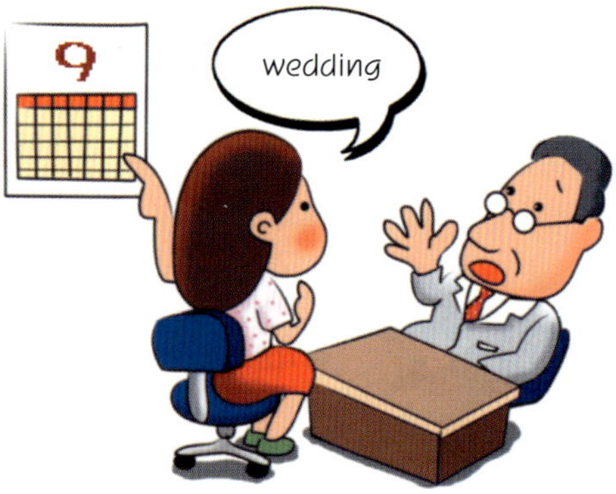

I'm getting married this Fall, can it be done before then?

I have had cases where patients would ask me to shorten the treatment period to less than a year because of employments, weddings, or other personal reasons. However, orthodontists cannot shorten the treatment period. Rather, the activities of the tissues that surround the teeth is the main factor for determining the duration of treatment. Just as the broken bones do not heal faster because you are hospitalized, it is equally applied to orthodontic treatment.

Even if the cells that form and resorb the bones keep at work without resting, the teeth will not move more than 2mm per month. This cannot be changed, because this is how God designed our bodies.

E. The Time that It Takes to Move the Teeth.

In the case of clustered tooth alignment as in the crowding, there may be no problems in the relationship between the upper and lower jaw. The appliance used for this type of treatment is usually adjusted once a month.

If a new appliance needs to be inserted or changed totally, then the visiting time for monthly treatment would take about an hour. But for normal adjustments, it takes about 20 minutes or so. The overall treatment period in this case generally would take up 2 years or so.

41. What is Considered Good Orthodontic Treatment?

A. Teeth Alignment in Balance with the Patient's Face

B. Hereditary Trend

C. Correlation between the Shape of the Face and Dental Arch

D. Short Treatment Period

E. Simple Appliances

F. Minimum Pain

G. Minimum Relapse

H. Unknown Origin Relapse

I. Duration of the Good Alignment of Teeth

J. Perfect Treatment Depends on the Patient

K. Patient's Stubbornness

L. Consistent Treatment

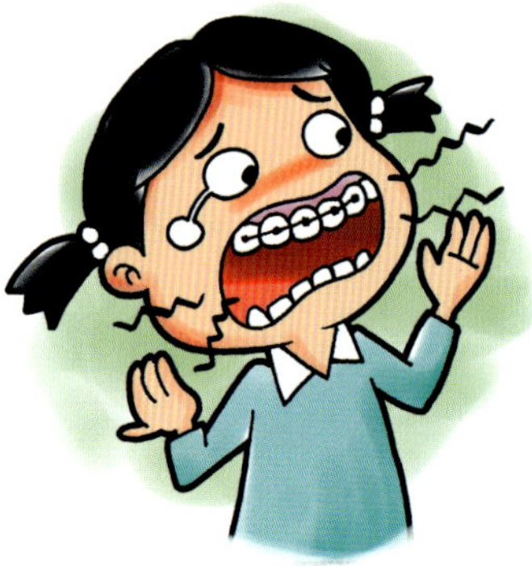

A. Teeth Alignment in Balance with the Patient's Face.

The orthodontist in charge will put great effort into determining the best teeth alignment for the individual patient. Examining the family photo for confirming hereditary trend, taking x-rays of the hand and wrist to confirm the growth spurt, comparing the configuration of the teeth arrangement(dental arch) with the facial type are all for that purpose.

B. Hereditary Trend

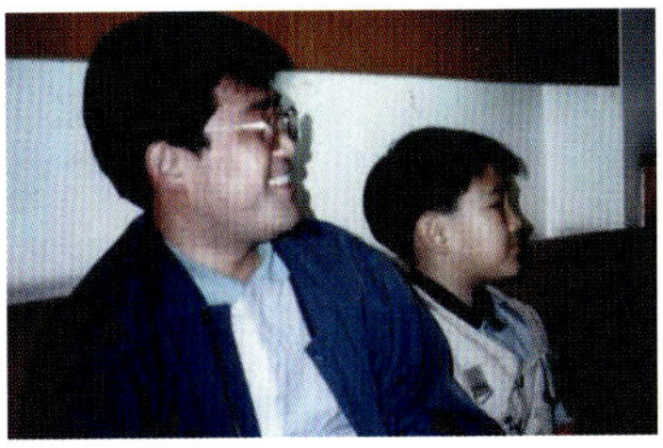

This photo shows hereditary similarities between son and father. The overall profile is similar to each other.

C. Correlation between the Shape of the Face and Dental Arch

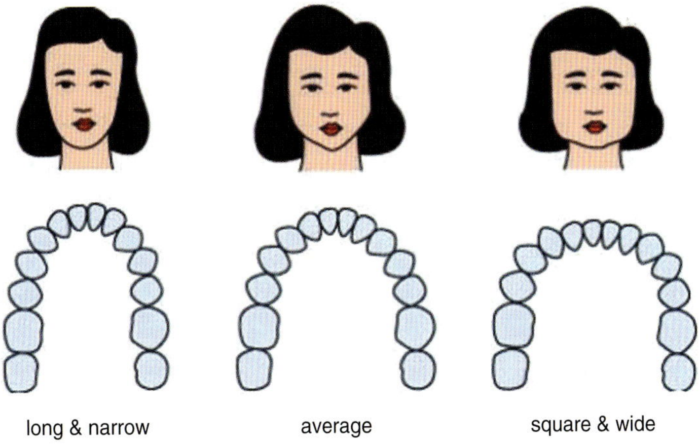

D. Short Treatment Period

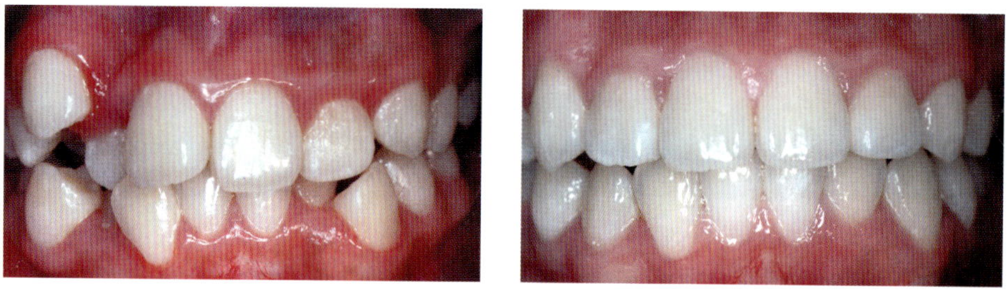

crowding treatment finished about 18 months

Because of her high canine teeth, each time she smiled, her lips got caught on it, and sometimes it would tear the inside of her mouth. She said that she had been going to her dentist for five years for treating this problem.

This kind of treatment usually takes about 2 years. If the treatment takes a very long time, it becomes a burden to the patient mentally and physically.

E. Simple Appliances

The multibanded bracket method used 20 years ago took all day just to place the brackets on the teeth. These days the band is used only on the molar, which receives the heaviest force. Even the band on molars are not used in some patients because of using mini pin for anchorage.

If the same effect can be achieved, it is best to use the simplest appliance. These days with the development of adhesive bonding materials, orthdontic appliances become very simple. If we used the same metallic bands that had been used in the old days on every patient, we would think that it is considered old-fashioned. If the appliance is simple, it is not only more comfortable for the patient, but it will look better.

F. Minimum Pain

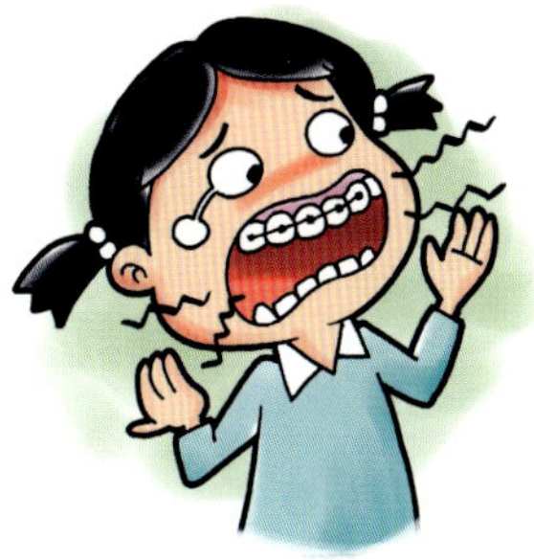

The best orthodontic treatment can be said if it has the least amount of pain. Fear of pain is a basic instinct for human beings. Although the orthodontist will do everything possible to bring about the least amount of pain, there is a tendency for increased pain in older patients and in situations where strong force is applied to the tooth. Pain during orthodontic treatment has decreased greatly due to the rapid development of medico-dental engineering. It will be a comfort to know that pain is a sign of the moving teeth.

G. Minimum Relapse

Relapse turns all the years of the patient's sufferings and doctor's efforts into nothing. Treatment is complete only when the treated teeth are in a stable state for a long time.

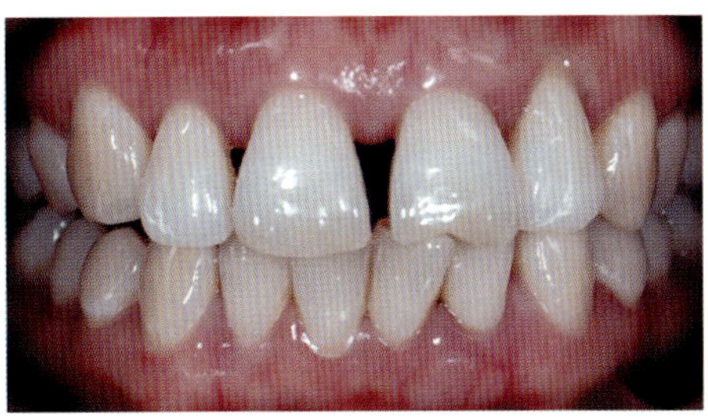

befrore treatment

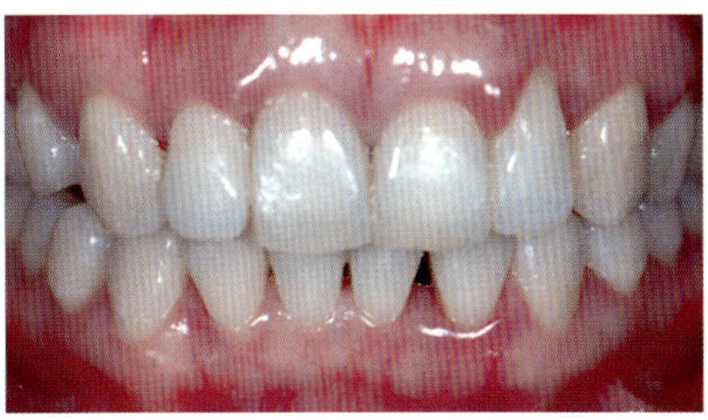

after treatment

Recently, a study has reported that the chin continues to grow although very small amounts, even when growing has completely stopped. That is, there are many patients who had good alignment of the upper front teeth when they were young, but as they grew older the upper front teeth started to gain space. This is because the lower jaw has grown outward, and pushes the upper front teeth out.

H. Unknown Origin Relapse

There are cases where the reasons for relapse are unknown. Slight relapse is inevitable. However, there is no need to worry since it is not a serious problem. It would not completely return to their original condition before the treatment, and it can be corrected easily with a simple appliances in a short period.

I. Duration of the Good Alignment of Teeth

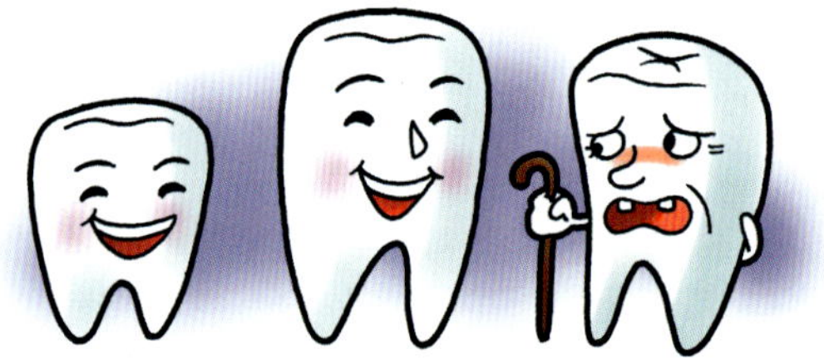

Another yardstick I would like to add is for how long the good and healthy alignment of teeth can be possessed . That is, it is better to have good teeth alignment from childhood than to have a good alignment for the first time as adults.

The beauty of youth with a bright smile and good alignment of teeth cannot be exchanged for anything in the world. If an adolescent is given more chances to prove himself because of the good impressions his appearance gives to others, then he will be confident in everything he does.

He will also have a positive outlook on life. This means that physical appearance plays a vital role in determining how a person views life.

J. Perfect Treatment Depends on the Patient

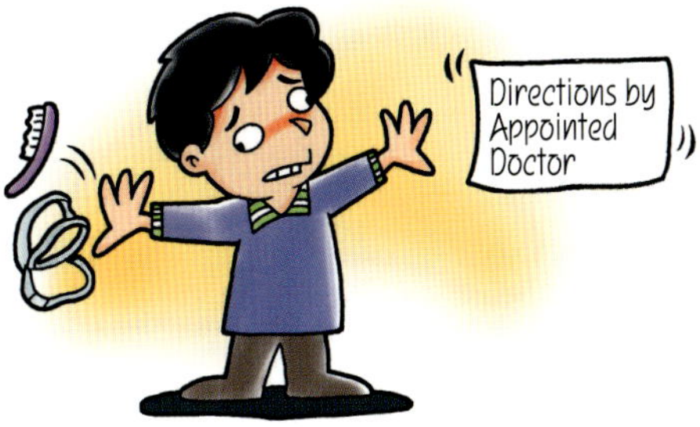

Many portions of the outcome of complete treatment is determined by the degree of the patient's cooperation. If the patient does not follow the orthodontist's instructions like brushing regularly, changing the rubber band daily, and wearing it all day long, then no matter how much the orthodontist tries, effective treatment cannot be obtained.

K. Patient's Stubbornness

In many cases, there are patients who, despite the orthodontist's explanation, request simple, quick, and inexpensive appliance even if it does not turn out to be a perfect result.

However, as many adults regret that they did not study harder during their youth, some patients may regret not following the orthodontist's suggestions. If the orthodontist satisfies patient's demand for financial aspects, the orthodontist is to blame, and I do not wish to satisfy these types of patient's desire on those terms.

L. Consistent Treatment

There are rare cases where patients change orthodontist during the middle of the treatment. From the orthodontist's perspective, there are problems in accepting consultations from a patient who had already received treatment at another dental clinic.

There are many techniques in orthodontic treatment and each orthodontist uses his own distinct technique, which he has mastered. Even if the technique is almost the same, the materials and instruments each orthodontist uses may differ. So, if an orthodontist treats a patient who has been initially receiving treatment elsewhere, there are bound to be minute differences in treating procedures.

Even if all of the patient's data is received from the previous orthodontist, the results will not be the same compared to the patient receiving treatment from the same orthodontist.

Also, the new orthodontist can use a different treatment method. In this case, another set of new x-rays will be needed and different appliances may be used. All of this will require the patient to pay redundant fees.

42. Orthodontic Treatment Fees

A. Diagnosis

B. Status of Doctor in Charge

C. Sensibility of Doctor in Charge

A. Diagnosis

A diagnostic materials are taken before starting orthodontic treatment. And then diagnosis and treatment plans are attained on the ground of diagnosis materials. A diagnosis contains important data that would determine the outcome of the treatment. Because the diagnosis is the most important process in orthodontic treatment, it forms a large share of the treatment fee.

But since the fees for X-rays, appraisal of growth and development, and study model analysis, and various other examination fees are also high, the fee only for the diagnosis seems comparatively low.

Of course, if you are only receiving a consultation for orthodontic treatment, you will only be charged for the visitation or consultation fee, and even if you did, that wouldn't be so expensive.

B. Status of the Doctor in Charge.

Medical fees are different from market prices where products are bought and sold.

Since orthodontic treatment is performed by an orthodontist with expert academic knowledge and skills in that field, the fee is not determined by only orthodontic materials used, but by the status of the doctor.

This is the same principle for a work of art by a famous artist, where the price is not determined by the materials such as brushes, and paints that are used.

C. Sensibility of the Doctor in Charge

The real value of the treatment is determined by good results, so it is not a wise method to choose an orthodontist based solely on the treatment fees.

Since orthodontic treatment requires expert knowledge and technique, it is not a good idea to ask for fees over the phone as like you would do as when purchasing goods. Making a decision based on informations over the phone is the same as buying a cheap product, only to regret the purchase later on. You can simply return products if you do not want; however, if you are unsatisfied with the treatment results, then you would not only have wasted precious time and money, but also it would be difficult to start treatment again for complete correction.

And in some cases, perfect treatment at the second time may be impossible. I am confident in saying that an able doctor provides treatment at reasonable fees.

43. Relapse After Orthodontic Treatment

A. Eruption of Wisdom Teeth and Late Growth

B. Fibrotomy

C. Postponement of Treatment Beginning

D. Retainer

E. Removable Type of Retainer

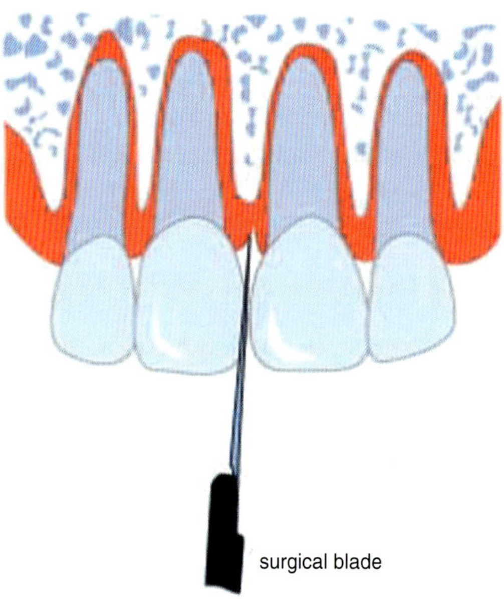

A. Eruption of Wisdom Teeth and Late Growth

Relapse can occur without any relation to the orthodontic treatment itself. After the treatment, the force from the eruption of the second molar or wisdom tooth may push the remaining teeth forward, thus disrupting the teeth alignment attained by long-term treatment. However, it can be corrected in a short period.

Also, a long and tilted lower jaw treated through surgery could relapse due to the late growth. Retreatment, even surgery again will be necessary if the lower teeth are severely tipped inward caused by excessive growth of lower jaw.

Even if, at the ages of 5 to 6 years, a chin cap is worn because of symptom of long and tilted lower jaw and the treatment is successful, but if it is neglected, growth will occur after 1~2 years causing long and tilted lower jaw to occur again. Therefore, even when normal alignment of teeth is obtained, the chin cap is continued to be worn during the night until the growth is ceased.

B. Fibrotomy

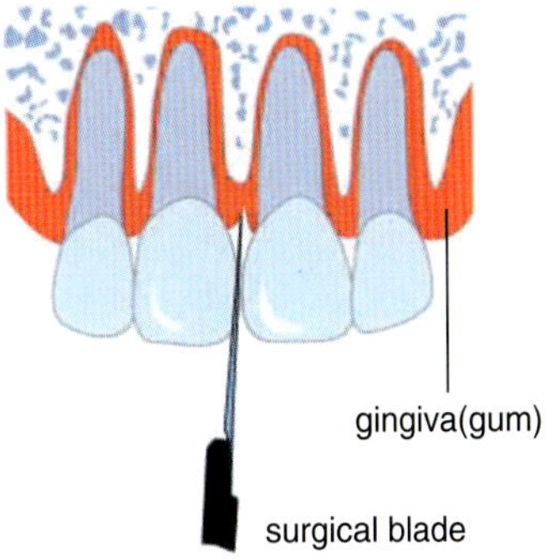

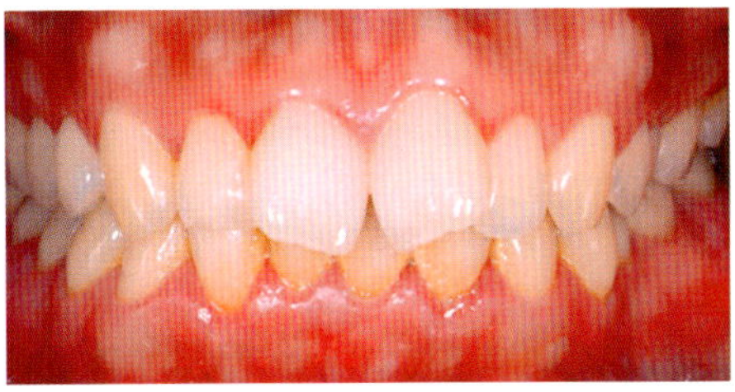

If the rotated tooth is corrected after treatment, a simple surgery to incise the gingiva (tooth gum) can be performed to prevent relapse. It is called "fibrotomy", but actually it is a simple procedure, which is painless and no bleeding, and full recovery is possible in a week.

C. Postponement of Treatment Beginning

Waiting for the treatment to start using brackets until the end of the growth period can be another way of minimizing the chances of relapse.

D. Retainer

Retainer is a device for keeping teeth alignment in position. Although the bonded brackets are completely removed after completion of treatment, teeth alignment is not in a stable condition.

If the teeth are neglected even for a day after removal of bonded brackets, the teeth can return toward their original condition. Therefore, they must be secured with a retainer immediately upon removal of the brackets.

A simple retainer is worn for about a year so that the teeth can adjust to their new environment. Retainers can be fixed or removable, but whatever form it may be, it will be simpler, less unseemingly, and less uncomfortable than the bonded brackets.

E. Removable Type of Retainer

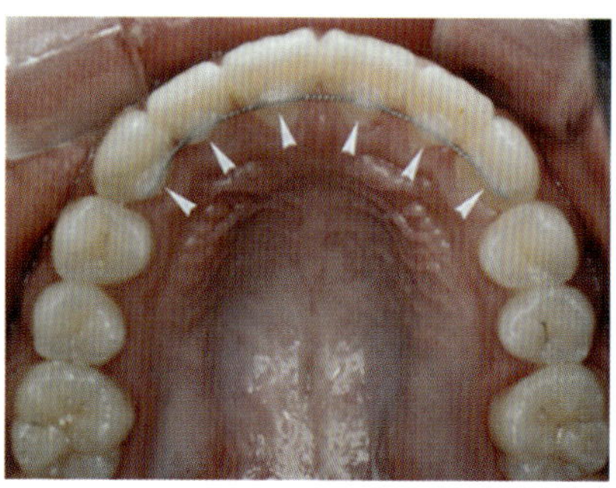

Fixed Type

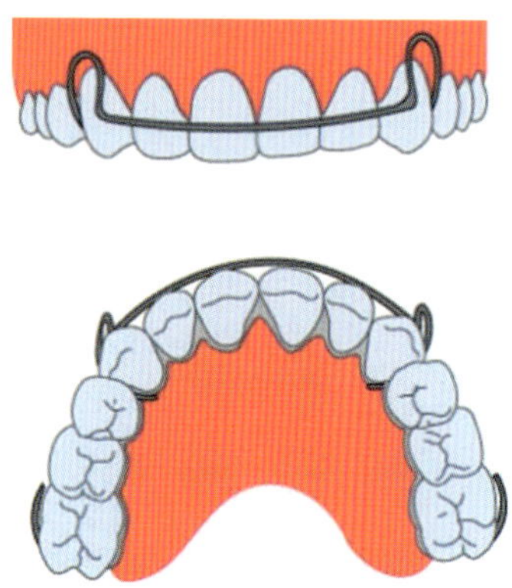

Removable Type

Fixed retainers are normally used for permanent corrections. After bonding fixed retainer, it is checked regularly at least twice a year.

The period for wearing a removable retainer differ according to the original state of malocclusion, but normally, for the first six months, it is worn at all times except when eating and brushing the teeth. Then, it will only be worn at night, and when there is absolutely no sign of relapse, it is totally removed.

While retainer is worn, the patient must visit the orthodontist once a month for the first year, then after that, 2~3 times a year using a comfortable day.

Epilogue

Korean society has been affected by globalization since its economical scale entered within 10th place in the world. Many foreigners who can speak English are living in Korea, and they also wish to get informed about orthodontic treatments. However, they often cannot fully get informations. I wrote this book because I thought that providing those informations was also part of responsibility of dentist who studied orthodontics.

I have never lived in English speaking countries before. But during years in Dentistry School, I won the third prize in English competitions for three consecutive times, and I once tried to go to the United States to study Orthodontics after the graduation. In that time, I studied English very hard. Thinking of writing English version of my book that explains orthodontic treatments might have been a reckless challenge. However, I have encountered many reckless challenges before such as entering dental college later than those of normal aged students, studying abroad when I did not have enough money at the age of 35 and etc. Because I previously experienced those hard times, I felt that it was worthwhile to write English book which was seemingly impossible.

Realizing it is way harder than I thought did not take much time as I tried to write accurate words and expressions. To do that, I looked up every word in the dictionary and I double-checked every grammar.

I noticed that I am not talented when I was writing this book. But after finishing this book, I now have higher self-esteem about writing in English which is not a mother-tongue language to me.

Elder son who is following my path to become a dentist in Matsumoto Dental University in Japan, and the younger son who is studying chemistry in the University of British Columbia, Canada helped me with changing my shamefully written English to more understandable sentences. The sentences became perfect after the help from my two sons, so that I put their names in this book as two members of translators.

When I was young I guided my two sons. But now their existences give a light to my remaining years and I am very satisfied. I believe that my wife and two sons will fulfill my life. Even though I have a tough time right now, I am as happy as can be because of my loving family.

I would like to take this opportunity to thank all the faculty members of Dentistry of Dankook University who taught with passion and sincerity. Also, I would like to thank professor Kawata, Tenshin, and Sou who helped and guided me during the Graduate School to become an orthodontic specialist during my study in Japan.

Last of all, I will give my passionate love to my wife whose sacrifices made my career as an orthodontist possible.

June 10, 2012. Ho-Sung, Lew

후일담

한국의 경제규모가 세계 10위안에 진입하면서 우리 사회 역시 세계화의 영향을 받게 되었다. 영어로 의사전달이 가능한 많은 외국인들이 한국에 살고 있고, 그들 역시 치아교정 치료에 관한 정보를 얻고 싶어 하지만 이에 관한 책이 없는 실정이다. 이런 사람들에게 치과교정에 관한 정보를 제공하는 것 역시 치과 교정학을 전공한 사람이 해야 할 일 중의 하나라는 생각 때문에 이 책을 쓰게 되었다.

영어권의 나라에서 살아본 적이 전혀 없지만 치과대학 재학 중 교내에서 실시한 영어 경시대회에 참가하여 연속 3회 3위에 입상한 경력도 있고, 미국 유학을 하려고 한 때 정열을 바쳐 영어 공부에 매달려 본 적은 있다. 치과교정 치료에 관한 영어책을 집필하려고 마음먹었던 것 자체가 무모한 도전이었는지도 모른다. 하지만 늦은 나이에 치과대학에 입학한 것, 경제적으로 넉넉지 않던 30 중반의 나이에 박사학위를 받기 위해 일본 유학을 떠났던 것도 무모한 도전이었기에 그 가치를 몸소 체험하기 위해 실행에 옮기게 되었다.

영문판 저서집필이 생각보다 훨씬 어려운 작업임을 깨닫는 데는 많은 시간이 걸리지 않았다. 정확한 표현을 만들려고 단어 하나하나 일일이 사전을 찾아가며 용법을 확인하며 문장을 만들어 갔다. 이번 책을 집필하면서 학문의 깊이가 없고, 재주가 없음을 다시금 뼈저리게 느끼게 되었지만, 60이 가까운 나이에 교정의로서 일을 하면서 모국어가 아닌 영어로 책을 썼다는 자부심 하나만은 가지게 되었다.

일본에서 대를 이어 치과의학을 공부하고 있는 장남, 캐나다 밴쿠버 UBC대학에서 화학을 전공하고 있는 차남이 치졸한 수준으로 쓰인 영어 문장을 읽기 쉽고, 이해하기 쉬운 문장으로 만들어 주었다. 두 아들의 힘을 빌려 완전한 번역이 되었기에 번역자의 명단에 넣었다.

어릴 때는 내가 두 아들을 인도하였지만 나이가 들다보니 이 두 아들이 내 여생의 길이 되어주고 빛을 주는 존재가 되는 것 같아 흡족하다. 앞으로도 나의 부족한 부분을 내 아내와 두 아들이 채워 주리라 믿기에 지금 삶이 고되긴 하지만, 더 없이 행복하다.

치과의사라는 직업을 가질 수 있도록 열과 성을 다해 지도해 주신 단국대학교 치과대학 교수님, 일본 유학중 치과교정과 전문 과정을 이수하도록 돌보아 주시고, 박사학위 과정을 끝낼 수 있도록 헌신적으로 도와주신 카와타 교수, 텐신 교수, 소 교수님께 심심한 감사를 드립니다.

마지막으로 치과교정전문의로서 지금의 위치에 설 수 있도록 물심양면으로 희생을 아끼지 않은 아내 권위숙에게 이 자리를 빌려 깊은 애정을 보냅니다.

2012년 6월 10일 내가 태어난 날 류 호 성

References

References

1. Jablonsky: Illustrated Dictionary of Dentistry. W.B. Saunders, 1982.
2. Proffit WR: Contemporary Orthodontics. St. Louis Mosby 3rd Edition, 2000.
3. Robert E. Moyers: Handbook of Orthodotntics. Year Book Medical Publishing, Inc 4th Edition, 1988.
4. Graber & Neuman: Removable Orthodontic Appliances. W.B. Saunders, 2nd Edition, 1984.
5. S.N. Bhaskar: Orban°Øs Oral Histology and Embriology. C.V. Mosby, 9th Edition, 1980.
6. R.M.H. McMainn et al: A Color Atlas of Head and Neck Anatomy. Wolfe Medical Publications Ltd., 1981.
7. JH Witzig et al: The Clinical Management of Basic Maxillofacial Orthopedic Appliances. Year Book Medical Publishing, Inc., 1987.
8. TM Graber, RL Vanarsdall, jr.: Orthodotntics Current Principles and Techniques. CV Mosby, 3rd Edition, 2000.
9. DH Enlow: Handbook of Facial Growth. WB Saunders, 2nd Edition, 1982.
10. S Ramfjord, Major M Ash: Occlusion. WB Saunders, 3rd Edition, 1983.
11. TM Graber, T. Rakosi, AG Petrovic: Dentofacial Orthopedics with Functional Appliances. C.V. Mosby, 2nd Edition, 1997.
12. JA Salzman: Orthodontics in Daily Pratice. JB Lippincott Company, 1st Edition 1974.
13. WJ Clark: Twin Block Functional Therapy. Mosby-Wolfe, 1995.
14. TM Graber: Orthodontics, Principles and Practice. WB Saunders, 3rd Edition, 1974.
15. EW Renfroe: Edgewise. Lea & Febiger, 1975.
16. FV Tenti: Atlas of Orthodontic Appliances, Fixed and Removable. Carvel, Italy, 1986.
17. JP Okeson: Fundamentals of Occlusion and Temporomandibular Disorders. CV Mosby, 1985.
18. TD Foster: A Textbook of Orthodontics. Blackwell Scientific Publications, 2nd Edition, 1982.
19. JC Bennet, RP McLaughlin: Orthodontic Management of the Dentition with the Preadjusted Appliance. Isis Medical Media, London, 1997.
20. RC Wheeler: Dental Anatomy, Physiology, and Occlusion, WB Saunders, 1974.
21. HS, Lew: A Beauty Made in Dental Clinic. Cyberdental, Seoul, Korea, 2005.

Index

Index

U

W

A Dentist Can Make You More Beautiful!

Myung Mun Publishing. Co.
#90, 63 Gil, Dapsimni-ro, Dongdaemun-gu,
Seoul, Korea
TEL. +82-2-2248-7586
FAX. +82-2-2248-0598
e-mail. mmayt@hanmail.net
Website. www.teethbook.co.kr
ISBN. 978-89-87037-98-1

First Edition by Ho-Sung, Lew, D.D.S., Ph.D.
Orthodontic Specialist

Printed in Korea

US $50